HOW TO MANAGE AND TREAT DIABETES WITH STARVATION TREATMENT

Exploring a sequence of stepped Diets

By

Bob Philz

TABLE OF CONTENTS

OVERVIEW.

Unquestionably, one of the most beneficial treatments for diabetes is the "starvation treatment," as promoted by Dr. Frederick M. Allen of the Rockefeller Institute Hospital. It has been used for several months at the Massachusetts General Hospital with great success. It is believed to be worthwhile to publish some of the diets and treatment details that have been employed there because a very careful control of the protein and carbohydrate intake is essential to the success of the treatment. When implementing the Allen therapy, there is need to consider grams of both carbohydrates and proteins; it isn't sufficient to only limit the patient's intake of starchy meals; but also needs to be aware of the patient's daily intake of these nutrients. Since calculating these dietary parameters might be difficult for a busy practitioner, the series of estimated diets provided here may be helpful. Of course, any good chemistry textbook will have the various tests for sugar, acetone, etc., but it is worth while to add them here for convenience and completeness. The majority of common foods are included in the food table.

Specifics of the therapy

To assess the extent of this diabetes treatment, a research was conducted such that the patient is kept on a regular diet for 48 hours following hospital admission. After that, he becomes starving and is only permitted to eat whiskey and black coffee. One ounce of whiskey is served with coffee every two hours starting at seven in the morning. up to 7:00 p.m. This provides approximately 800 calories. The whiskey provides a few calories and makes the patient more comfortable during the starvation process; it is not a necessary component of the treatment. If whiskey is not preferred, one may substitute it with bouillon or any other clear soup. It is not necessary to limit the water consumption. If there is significant evidence of acidosis, as shown by strong acetone and diacetic acid reactions in the urine or a strong acetone odor on the breath, soda bicarbonate may be administered, two drachms every three hours. Generally speaking, though, this is not required at all, and fasting poses no risk of causing a coma. In fact, this is the most significant point that Dr. Allen has made during his course of treatment. Initially, it was believed that it was ideal to keep patients in bed for the duration of the fast, but it is undeniably true that most patients fare better and achieve sugar-free status faster if they are active and engage in moderate activity for at least some of the day. Until there is no more sugar in the urine, starvation is maintained. (Of course, the daily weight and urine examinations are recorded.) The sugar disappears quickly: if it was 5 or 6 percent, it may drop to 2 percent after the first starvation day, and the patient may be completely sugar-free or may have.2 or.3 percent the following day. of sweets. On rare occasions, it could take longer. We have only fasted a patient for a maximum of four days, but in some stubborn situations, we have starved patients for ten or eleven days without negative outcomes. The patients have an amazing ability to withstand malnutrition; we have never observed any negative consequences from it. It's possible that you'll lose three or four pounds, but that's not significant. In fact, according to Allen, most diabetics should aim for a moderate weight loss. If a patient is moderately obese and weighs 180 pounds, for example, he may still excrete a small amount of sugar even if he consumes very little in the way of carbohydrates. However, if he loses weight and drops to 170 or 160 pounds, he can easily remain sugar-free on the same diet. It is imperative that a fat diabetic lose weight and maintain it there.

There was no consistent behavior of the acetone and diacetic acid output during fasting observed; in certain instances, it was observed the acetone bodies to vanish, and in other instances, we have observed them to emerge when they were absent previously.

It's not always necessary to be alarmed by their appearance. Estimating the ammonia in the urine can help determine the degree of acidosis present, and the straightforward chemical approach below makes this process easy to accomplish. A significant amount of acidosis is present if the 24-hour ammonia output exceeds 3 or 4 grams; anything less than this is not noteworthy. The ratio of total urine nitrogen to ammonia, the amount of acetone, diacetic acid, and oxy-butyric acid expelled, and the carbon dioxide tension of the alveolar air are more precise ways to measure the degree of acidosis. However, these are a bit too complex for routine clinical application.

After the patient stops eating sugar, his diet is changed to include just "5% vegetables," or veggies with about 5% carbohydrate. Boil these vegetables three times, changing the water between each boil. They thereby cut their carbohydrate content in half, most likely. If preferred, a modest quantity of fat in the form of butter may be consumed along with this veggie diet. These green vegetables contain a significant amount of carbohydrates; if the patient eats to his heart's content, he may consume as much as 25 or 30 grams, which is far too much; the first day following starvation, the patient's carbohydrate intake should not exceed 15 grams. The vegetable diets shown here are in Tables No. 1 and No. 2. Typically, diets 1 or 2 are administered to the patient for a duration of one day, or two days in the case of a particularly severe condition. Following the vegetable day, protein and fat levels rise while carbohydrate levels remain unchanged (diets 2, 3, and 4). Although there is no hard and fast rule for how long a patient should follow a certain diet, we generally don't recommend really low diets like 2, 3, and 4 for longer than a day or two at a time. Increases in the diet should be made very gradually, and it is not a good idea to increase the amount of protein and carbohydrates at the same time because it's important to determine which is more problematic. Although the protein consumption may increase more quickly than the carbohydrate intake, too much protein is a major factor in the development of glycosuria, thus it needs to be monitored just as carefully as the carbohydrate intake. If at all possible, adults should receive one gram of protein for every kilogram of body weight; youngsters should receive 1.5 to 2 grams. You'll see that the diets that follow have much less fat in them than what is often prescribed for diabetes. This is due to two factors: first, we want to prevent weight gain in our adults with diabetes; second, if fat consumption is kept low, acidosis is much easier to treat. It is relatively simple to add fat in the form of butter, milk, or bacon if the fat values recommended in the diets are discovered to be too low for any particular situation. The majority of people function effectively on roughly 30 calories per kilogram of body weight; four-year-olds require 75 calories per kilogram, eight-year-olds require 60, and twelve-year-olds require 50.

We return to a lower diet if sugar is detected in the urine while the diet is being raised; if this doesn't work, we begin another starving day and increase the diet more gradually. However, if the diet is increased very gradually, sugar won't show up. Pushing an average case is not a good idea; if the patient is on a decent diet, say 50 percent protein, 50 percent carbohydrate, and 150 percent fat, and is doing well with no glycosuria, then it is not a good idea to increase the diet any further. Some of these diets appear to have quite low calorie intakes, yet it's amazing how well most patients function on 1500 or 2000 calories.

It will be evident that there are three steps to the treatment:

1. The starvation stage, during which the patient is starting to avoid sugar.
2. The phase in which the diet is progressively increased to the point of tolerance. A daily weight log and daily urine

examinations should be conducted during the first two phases. Of course, the patient should be under the doctor's direct observation during these two phases. If at all feasible, it is best to send a patient home with a diet that is somewhat below his tolerance.

3. The stationary phase, during which the food is maintained at the same quantity. The patient is at his house, carrying on with his activities. It's possible that most patients will learn how to test their own urine, which they should do every other day. The patient should return to a lesser diet if there is sugar in the urine; if this method is not successful in making him sugar-free, he should once more go without food. Whether or not the urine has sugar, a semi-starvation day of 150 grams of vegetables once a week is beneficial for maintaining the patient well within the margin of safety and serving as a reminder that he is following a tight diet.

Engaging in regular exercise is crucial for diabetics since it improves their ability to use carbohydrates.

The patient must carefully measure out everything and follow the instructions exactly if they want this treatment to be successful. Meat in particular needs to be weighed.

You'll notice that the diets' caloric intake occasionally differs somewhat from the amounts of protein, fat, and carbohydrates. The reason for this is that the calories have been provided in round amounts for convenience's sake; it doesn't matter if there are five or ten calories.

The following are the main ideas that Allen's treatment highlights:

- Unlike the old treatment of progressively reducing the amount of carbohydrates, starving a diabetic patient for two or three days almost invariably results in sugar-free status, saving a significant amount of time. Starvation is not hazardous.
- Maintaining their weight is not ideal for all diabetics. If ten, fifteen, or even twenty pounds are taken off the weight of some instances, they might do far better.
- To stop glycosuria from recurring after deprivation, the diet must be increased very gradually.
- It is important to recognize that too much protein can cause glycosuria and too much fat can cause ketonuria. Therefore, consuming less protein and fat than normal is necessary when managing diabetes.

Case Studies.

For the sake of illustration, it is deemed worthwhile to incorporate a few case studies. While the children received treatment at the Children's Hospital, the adults received care at Massachusetts General Hospital.

For every case, two charts are maintained: one is a food chart that lists the various food items and their daily amounts, together with the protein, carbohydrate, fat, and calorie values for each; the other is a more general chart (see below) that visually depicts the case's development.

The first three cases, which ranged from 0.1% to 0.2% of sugar, were first treated using the outdated technique of progressively cutting back on carbohydrate consumption. These cases were never able to be made sugar-free. They responded quickly to the new medication and were released sugar-free.

Case One (A 64 year Old)

64-year-old woman with two years of diabetes. She had been receiving a diet consisting of 50 grams of carbohydrates and 50 grams of protein from the outpatient department when she was sent in. She was excreting 8 grams of sugar daily from her diet, and her urine was exhibiting quite severe reactivity to acetone and diacetic acid. She released 3 grams of sugar daily when the ward's carbohydrate intake was reduced to 30 grams. She reported having excruciating vulvae pruritus. Following sixteen days of treatment, she continued to consume between 0.1% and 0.2% of sugar daily. Following the initiation of Allen's treatment, she went without sweets for four days, following a diet consisting of 20 grams of carbohydrates, 30 grams of protein, and 150 grams of fat. The itch had subsided. She then displayed 1.5% of sugar and the protein was increased to 80 grams and the carbohydrate to 20 grams. It is crucial to remember not to elevate the protein too soon. We were unaware of this in our previous cases.

After two days of hunger, two days of vegetables, and a more cautious increase in the diet, she was discharged without consuming any sugar. Her eating regimens were:

December 12.

- Twenty grams of carbs.
- Thirty grams of protein.
- 150 grams to 1500 calories of fat. Absence of glycosuria.

December 15.

- Thirty grams of carbs.
- Thirty grams of protein.
- 200 grams or 2000 calories of fat. Absence of glycosuria.

December 20.

- Thirty grams of carbs.
- 40 grams of protein.
- 180 grams of fat = 2000 calories. Absence of glycosuria.

December 26.

- Forty grams of carbs.
- 40 grams of protein.
- 180 grams of fat = 2000 calories. Absence of glycosuria.

December 30.

- Fifty grams of carbs.
- 50 grams of protein.
- 180 grams of fat = 2000 calories. Absence of glycosuria.

Arrived hospital weighing 119 pounds and at discharge, 116 pounds in weight.

Case Two (A 49 Year Old)

At admission, a 49-year-old Jew had 175 grams of sugar (5.5%), a small amount of acetone, and no diacetic acid. After receiving treatment for three weeks using the previous approach, he reduced his daily intake of sugar to 3 to 8 grams and increased his intake of protein to 50 grams. We were unable to eliminate the last traces of sugar using the previous procedure.

Two days of hunger preceded the initiation of the Allen therapy. He had no sugar on the second, but the next day, he had 2.6 grams of sugar along with 12 grams of carbohydrates and 40 grams of protein. (This was one of the first times the diet was increased too rapidly following fasting.) He continued to avoid sweets after two vegetable days and one more starvation day, and the diet was gradually increased to 45 grams of protein and 30 grams of carbohydrates, or roughly 2000 calories. sugar-free discharged on this diet.

109 pounds was the entrance weight and at discharge, 110 pounds in weight.

Case Three (A 35 Year Old)

On December 28,1914, a 35-year-old guy with serious diabetes entered. He had spent a month in the hospital the July before, and the previous treatment approach would never have allowed him to go sugar-free. He was releasing 2.5% of sugar (135 grams) daily upon admission, and his acetone and diacetic acid tests were overwhelmingly high. He was sugar-free after two starvation days, however we erred by not using twice-boiled veggies on his vegetable day following fasting. He so consumed roughly 30 grams of carbohydrates on this particular day, and over the next four days, he displayed 0.2% to 1% of sugar. He was given another day of hunger and stopped eating sweets. This time, he was fed very little vegetables—just enough twice-boiled veggies to feed him with roughly 15 grams of carbs. Following this, the diet was gradually increased. After abstaining from sugar for three weeks, he was released.

- Twenty grams of carbs.
- 40 grams of protein.
- 200 grams of fat.
- He never took in more calories than 2200.

139 pounds was the entry weight and 138 pounds was his weight upon release.

These three cases were the first ones attempted, and in all three it was erred by increasing the diet too quickly, either by permitting an excessive amount of vegetables on the vegetable day or by increasing the protein too soon afterward. There was no longer any issue with the subsequent cases as we gained more experience.

Case Four (A 48 Year Old)

On January 14, 1915, a 48-year-old Greek male who had been diabetic for two months arrived with a moderate acetone response and 3.8% (65 grams) of sugar. At the entry, there was no diacetic reaction. After going without sweets for a day, he was put on famine for an additional day before beginning the regular regimen of eating vegetables. Moderate levels of diacetic acid started to show up in the urine after the third day and persisted. The daily ammonia increased to 2.6 grams from 0.7 grams, and then fluctuated between 0.3 and 1.5 grams. Absence of acidosis symptoms.

January 18.

- Fifteen grams of carbohydrates.
- 25 grams of protein.
- 150 grams of fat is 1360 calories. Absence of glycosuria.

January 20.

- Fifteen grams of carbohydrates.
- 25 grams of protein.
- 200 grams of fat, or 1571 calories. Absence of glycosuria.

January 24.

- 25 grams of carbohydrates.
- 35 grams of protein.

- 200 grams of fat = 1760 calories. Absence of glycosuria.

January 26.

- 35 grams of carbohydrates.
- 40 grams of protein.
- 200 grams of fat, or 1838 calories. Absence of glycosuria.

January 29.

- 45 grams of carbohydrates.
- 50 grams of protein.
- 200 grams of fat = 2194 calories. Absence of glycosuria.

January 31.

- Fifty grams of carbs.
- 60 grams of protein.
- 200 grams of fat = 2347 calories. Absence of glycosuria.

Discharged on this diet, sugar-free, on February 1, 160 pounds was the entrance weight and Weight of 156 pounds at discharge.

This was not a serious case, and the patient took the medication quite well.

Case Five (A 59 Year Old)

On January 16, 1915, a 59-year-old woman who had been diabetic for two years passed 2.6% of her sugar in her urine without experiencing any acetone or diacetic acid responses. intense vulvae pruritus. Two days of hunger; on the second day, no sugar was consumed and the pruritus vanished.

January 21.

- Fifteen grams of carbohydrates.
- 25 grams of protein.
- 150 grams of fat = 1595 calories. Absence of glycosuria.
- The diet was gradually increased after this point till on

January 30th, she started to receive

- 35 grams of carbohydrates.
- 45 grams of protein.
- 200 grams of fat = 2156 calories.

After spending two weeks in the wards, she was allowed to have no sweets and was then released to the out-patient department.

Upon entry, 135 pounds in weight and at discharge, 133 pounds in weight.

Case Six (A 52 Year Old)

On January 10, 1915, a 52-year-old man entered with 1% of sugar. He was seen for hypertension and arteriosclerosis, and the normal urine test revealed the presence of sugar. After a few days on a home diet, his blood sugar level increased to 3.5%. Not even diacetic acid or acetone. He stopped eating sugar after two days of fasting and kept on doing so while the diet was gradually increased. He was denied sweets for eighteen days while in the ward, and on February 6th, he followed a diet of

- 60 grams of carbohydrates.
- 60 grams of protein.
- 200 grams of fat = 2280 calories.

On February 7, there was an increase in protein to 80 grams and a 0.2% sugar level in the urine. After that, the protein was cut to 60 grams, and he was allowed to go off the regimen without consuming any sweets.

In this instance, a moderate amount of acetone started to develop and continued after hunger. Absence of acidosis symptoms. The daily ammonia levels ranged from 0.3 to 1.0 grams.

- 160 pounds was the entrance weight.
- 156 pounds following three weeks of treatment.
- Max calories consumed: 2525.

Case Seven (A 25 Year Old)

On January 20, 1915, a 25-year-old man who had been diabetic for eight months was admitted with a 6.6% (112 gram) sugar level and highly positive results for acetone and diacetic acid. He was sugar-free after two starving days, and he actually gained three pounds at that time (perhaps as a result of water retention).

The following was then added to his diet:

January 24.

- Fifteen grams of carbohydrates.
- 25 grams of protein.
- 150 grams of fat. Absence of glycosuria.

January 26.

- Twenty grams of carbs.
- 35 grams of protein.
- 175 grams of fat. Absence of glycosuria.

January 29.

- Twenty grams of carbs.
- 45 grams of protein.
- 200 grams of fat. Absence of glycosuria.

January 31.

- Thirty grams of carbs.
- 45 grams of protein.
- 200 grams of fat. Absence of glycosuria.

His daily ammonia was 1.7 grams at the entrance; during the days of hunger, it decreased to 0.3 grams. With the exception of three days, the acetone was slightly stronger than it was at the entrance.

He weighed 127 pounds on February 5, having gained seven pounds since entering, and remained sugar-free as he had been for the previous two weeks. He never got more than 2150 calories.

This was a really good example; the carbohydrate could have been increased to fifty or sixty grams, but he was responding so well that we thought it would be foolish to proceed.

Diabetes is probably much more severe in youngsters than it is in adults. However, in the few instances that the Children's Hospital has used the fasting treatment, the outcomes have been excellent in terms of making the youngster sugar-free. While weight loss is a crucial component of treatment for most adults with diabetes, it does not seem as desired for the majority of diabetic children who are small and weak and do not have excess weight to drop. Remarkably well, the few treated youngsters have survived famine. Although it is too early and we haven't seen enough kids treated with this technique to determine its potential impact on the disease's trajectory, it is undeniably effective in making them sugar-free.

Case Eight (A 12 Year Old)

M. M., a 12-year-old girl, arrived at the Children's Hospital on April 1, 1915. She had been on a standard diet at home and had likely had diabetes for six months. Charts on pages 31–36 are shown.

She had 8.7% sugar on the ward's regular diet and no acetone or diacetic acid. 52-1/4 pounds; she was an extremely slender, weak girl. After two days of starvation, she consumed around 1-1/2 ounces. of whiskey daily with a cup of black coffee.

On the first day of the fast, the urine's sugar level dropped to 2.3% and there was a faint acetone traces. She had a little acetone reaction and was sugar-free on the second day of hunger. Soda bicarbonate was not provided. She went through two pounds of malnutrition. Following her sugar-free conversion, her diets were as follows:

5 April.

- One and a half ounces of whiskey.
- Five grams of protein.
- Twelve grams of carbs.
- Seven grams of fat. Absence of glycosuria.
- 213. Calories.

April 6.

- One and a half ounces of whiskey.
- 26 grams of protein.
- 18 grams of carbohydrates.
- 46 grams of fat. Absence of glycosuria.
- 768 calories.

April 8.

- One and a half ounces of whiskey.
- 45 grams of protein.
- 22 grams of carbohydrates.
- 72 grams of fat. Absence of glycosuria.
- Ten hundred fifty calories.

April 9.

- One and a half ounces of whiskey.
- 58 grams of protein.
- 36 grams of carbohydrates.
- 86 grams of fat. Absence of glycosuria.
- Thirteen hundred nine calories.

Her diet was steadily increased after this, and on **April 16** she started taking the following:

- Four pieces of bacon.
- Two tablespoons of oatmeal.
- Two slices of bread.
- One ounce of meat.
- Five tablespoons of cabbage.
- Five tablespoons of spinach.
- Pick five tablespoons of string beans.

- Two ounces of butter.

This was computed to

- 64 grams of protein.
- 63 grams of carbohydrates.
- 113 grams of fat.
- 1546 calories.

She excreted.40% sugar while following this diet.

The bread was reduced to a single piece the following day, and her sugar vanished. She was eating meat and veggies on April 20 and consuming 4 tablespoons of oatmeal and 1 piece of bread without added sugar. This diet included:

- 63 grams of protein.
- 59 grams of carbohydrates.
- 112 grams of fat.
- 1521 calories.

Using the same diet, she expelled 1.1% of the sugar on April 21. Her porridge was reduced to 2 tablespoons the following day, providing her with roughly 10 grams less of carbohydrates. Absence of glycosuria. Sugar-free on **April 24**, she was released from

- 63 grams of protein.
- fifty grams of carbs.
- 112 grams of fat.
- 1510 calories.

Her urine had only a small amount of acetone and no diacetic acid at all. She gained some of the two pounds she lost during the starvation back, so when she was released from the hospital, her weight had decreased by only one pound. She has been going to the out-patient department every two weeks, and she looks to be in excellent health. She has never had any acetone, sugar, or diacetic acid in her urine. Her diet remains essentially the same as it was when she was discharged from the hospital. A rather easy case that improved quickly with therapy. Can she grow and develop on a diet that will prevent her from consuming sugar?

Case Nine (A 3 and Half Year Old)

A 3-1/2-year-old female, arrived on April 7, 1915, having dropped weight gradually over the previous month and experiencing extreme thirst and polyuria. had followed a standard diet at home. The boy was in a semi-conscious state at admission, and there were significant acetone, sugar, and diacetic acid reactions in his urine. She was placed on a milk diet with grated soda bicarbonate for the first twelve hours. xxx every two hours, and the following day was spent in starvation, taking one drachm of whiskey and bicarbonate soda orally and intrarectally. After starving for one day, she passed away. The girl was nearly moribund and in a coma when she was admitted to the hospital, thus it is difficult to consider this a valid test case for the starvation treatment. No matter what kind of care they receive, diabetics—old or young—rarely awaken from comas.

Case Ten (A Six Year Old)

A six-year-old boy, arrived on April 29, 1915. His diabetes was unknown for a while; it wasn't identified until the day of admission. A thin, malnourished-looking boy. He would first consume very little, excreting 5.7% of sugar, a moderate quantity of acetone, and a very little trace of diacetic acid on a ward diet consisting of 31 grams of protein, 73 grams of carbohydrates, and 20 grams of fat.

Starving, he drank 1-1/2 ounces of whiskey on May 2. It just took him a single day of starving to become sugar-free. His diet was increased progressively until May 7, when he was consuming 32 grams of protein, 33 grams of carbohydrates, and 75 grams of fat. He was also not consuming any sugar and was not taking acetone or diacetic acid. On May 9, he consumed 45 grams of carbohydrates and eliminated 40 percent of the sugar. It was reduced to 40 grams on May 10 and he passed out 2.2% sugar.

It was reduced to 20 grams on May 11 and he stopped eating sugar. He continued on this diet until June 8, when he was released from the hospital.

- Three tablespoons of string beans.
- Four tablespoonfuls of spinach.
- Four pieces of bacon.
- Two ounces of butter.
- Three eggs.
- Half a slice of bread.
- Two tablespoons of cereal.
- Three ounces of meat.
- 63 grams of protein.
- 31 grams of carbohydrates.
- 113 grams of fat.
- 1402 calories.

He had significant levels of acetone and small levels of diacetic acid in his urine for the first few days following admission, but they were gone throughout the remainder of his hospital stay. He weighed 31-1/2 pounds upon admission, 32-1/2 pounds upon discharge, and he did not lose weight while starving.

On two occasions, on July 31 and October 16, 1915, he was monitored in the out-patient department and maintained on a diet that was essentially the same. His urine only contained a trace amount of acetone and sugar. On November 9, his mother brought him in, stating that, although he had been eating well before, he had lost it. The boy's look was much the same as it had been the entire time, but his mother was told to get him into the wards right away so that he could be closely monitored for a few days. She promised to bring him in to stay the next day, but she wouldn't let him go. After she got him home, he unexpectedly fell into a coma and passed away that evening. This was a really terrible conclusion to a case that appeared to be quite satisfactory. Given the boy's mother's exceptional attention to detail and intelligence, it is quite likely that all dietary instructions were followed to the letter.

He must have suddenly gotten a severe acidosis because he had never displayed any symptoms of one.

Case Eleven (A 11 Year Old)

On November 3, 1915, an 11-year-old girl, was admitted to the Children's Hospital. She'd had diabetes for a good part of the year. She excreted 6.9% of sugar on a home diet with roughly 90 grams of carbohydrates, and her urine showed moderate responses to acetone and diacetic acid.

She went three days without food starting on Nov. 5. After going without food for three days, her blood sugar levels decreased to 3.5% on the first day, 1.1% on the second, and zero on the third. Her urine also contained somewhat more acetone than usual but less diacetic acid. Her diet was changed as follows after that:

November 8.

- Nine grams of protein.
- Twenty grams of carbs.
- Nine grams of fat. Absence of glycosuria.
- 200 calories.
- November 9.
- Seven grams of protein.
- Fifteen grams of carbohydrates.
- 35 grams of fat. Absence of glycosuria.
- There are 415 calories.

November 10.

- 17 grams of protein.
- Fifteen grams of carbohydrates.
- 55 grams of fat. Absence of glycosuria.
- 625 calories.

November 11.

- 38 grams of protein.
- Twenty grams of carbs. Absence of glycosuria.
- 88 grams of fat.
- 1055 calories.

On **November 13**, she added two tablespoons of oatmeal to her diet, bringing her total carbohydrate consumption to roughly thirty grams. That day, her sugar level was.6%. After being starved for thirty minutes, she resumed her sugar-free diet.

She took 40 grams of protein, 20 grams of carbohydrates, 90 grams of fat, 1080 calories, and no glycosuria on November 16.

On **November 17**, her diet consisted of 43 grams of protein, 25 grams of carbohydrates, 140 grams of fat, 1538 calories, and.5% sugar. After the amount of carbohydrates was reduced to 15 grams and maintained there for three days, she was fasted once more on November 21 and promptly stopped excreting sugar. Following this, her diet was increased until November 30, when she was discharged, consuming 48 grams of protein, 15 grams of carbohydrates, 110 grams of fat, 1280 calories, and no sweets for the previous nine days.

She weighed 56 pounds at admission, 54 pounds upon release, and lost 4 pounds due to malnutrition, which she partially gained back. She was barely maintaining her weight on the diet she was following at the time of her discharge. She never passed much acetone or diacetic acid, and the urine had only the tiniest amounts of these when she was released.

It is not advisable to increase the diet as quickly as it did in this instance, but due to unique circumstances, she had to leave the hospital as soon as possible, therefore her diets were increased a little sooner than they usually would have been.

Inspection of The Poo.

Instructions for Gathering 24-Hour Urine.

- Vacate the bladder by 7 a.m. and discard it.
- After this, save all pee passed until seven in the morning. the following day. At precisely seven in the morning, pass the pee and add it to what has already been passed.

Sugar Tests that Are Qualitative.

Fehling's Test: Boil for approximately 4 c.c. of Fehling's solution in a test tube, and then gradually add the same volume of urine—a few drops at a time—until the Fehling's boils after each addition.

Sugar is shown as a yellow or crimson precipitate.

Practically speaking, this is a useful test that we always utilize when monitoring a diabetic's daily pee.

Benedict's Test: Up to 5 c.c. Add eight drops of the urine to be tested to Benedict's[2] reagent. After boiling for one to two minutes, the liquid is let to cool naturally. Depending on the amount of sugar available, a red, yellow, or green precipitate is produced when dextrose is present. Due to precipitated urates, the solution may stay completely clear or become slightly turbid in the absence of sugar.

Fehling's test is less sensitive than this one.

Fehling's solution is made in this manner:

- ❖ 84.65 grams of copper sulphate solution. About 500 c.c. of copper sulfate dissolved in water.

❖ 125 grams of alkaline tartrate solution. of 178 grams and potassium hydroxide. About 500 c.c. of Rochelle salt dissolved in water.

When it's time to utilize them, these solutions are combined in equal amounts and stored in different bottles.

The components of Benedict's answer are as follows:

- 17.8 g of copper sulphate.
- 178.0 grams of sodium citrate.
- One kilogram of anhydrous sodium carbonate.
- raised the water's c.c. to 1000.
- Measurements of Sugar Content.

(1) The Fermentation Test: This is the most basic quantitative test for sugar and has a good enough degree of accuracy for use in clinical settings. The procedure is as follows: 100 c.c. and the specific gravity of the 24° urine are measured. portion of it into a flask, and then broke up and added a quarter of a yeast cake. After that, the flask is placed in a warm area that is roughly body temperature and left there for the night. A sample of the fermenting urine is tested for sugar the next morning. The urine is created up to 100 c.c. if there is no sugar present. (to account for the evaporated water) and repeat the specific gravity measurement. The amount of sugar in the urine is calculated by multiplying the number of specific gravity points lost by.23.

(2) Benedict's Test: This is the most accurate quantitative test for dextrose (except from polariscopic examination, which is too complex for daily use).

The procedure is as follows: Measure using a 25 c.c. pipette. Transfer 5 or 10 grams of Benedict's solution into a porcelain dish. of solid sodium bicarbonate, bring to a boil, and then pour the boiling mixture into the urine until a white precipitate develops.

The urine should then be added more gradually until the remaining traces of blue are gone. It is necessary to dilute the urine to a minimum of 10 c.c. will have to provide the quantity of sugar that the 25 c.c. reagent has the ability to oxidize.

Multiplying five by the total amount of c.c. of pee run-in, which is equivalent to 1%. of sweets.

The following is how Benedict's quantitative solution is made: dissolve 9.0 grams. of copper sulfate in one hundred cc. pure water. (The weight of the copper sulphate needs to be quite precise.) Dissolve 50 gm. 100 grams of anhydrous sodic carbonate. 65 grams of sodic citrate. in 250 c.c. of potassium sulphocyanate. of purified water.

Slowly pour the copper solution into the citrate solution that is alkaline. Then, without losing any of the mixture, pour the mixture into the flask until it reaches 500 c.c.; 25 c.c. 50 mgm less of this solution is used. 52 milligrams of dextrose. 67 mgm of levulose. of lactose.

Test for Acetone: Up to 5 c.c. Add a sodium nitro prusside crystal to a test tube containing pee. Add glacial acetic acid to acidify, shake for a second, and then add ammonium hydrate to make alkaline. Acetone is indicated by a purple hue.

Test for Diacetic Acid: Up to 5 c.c. Add an excess of a 10% ferric chloride solution to a test tube containing pee. Diacetyl red is an indicator of diacetic acid.

Ammonia Quantitative Test.

up to 25 c.c. add five c.c. of pee. About two to three drops of phenolphthalein in a saturated potassium oxalate solution.

Run in to a light pink tint from a burette decinormal sodic hydrate. Next, include five c.c. of formalin (commercial 40%) and titrate to the same hue once more.

Every c.c. = one c.c. of the decinormal alkali utilized in the last titration. of.0017 grams, or n/10 ammonia. of ammonia. Increase this by the quantity of c.c. The sodic hydrate employed in the previous titration, n/10, provides the ammonia grams in 25 c.c. pee.

It should be noted that both the formalin and the potassium oxalate need to be neutral to phenolphthalein.

One kilogram equals two pounds.

One calorie is equal to the amount of heat required to increase one kilogram of water's temperature by one degree Celsius.

9.3 calories are in 1 gram of fat.

Protein grams equal 4.1 calories.

4.1 calories per gram of carbohydrates.

DIETS.

All of the vegetables included in the following diet tables are boiled, with the exception of lettuce, cucumbers, celery, and raw tomatoes. They are boiled three times in very low-carb diets. The analyses for boiling veggies have been used if the figures could be obtained. It is predicted that when vegetables like cabbage and carrots are chopped into small pieces and cooked sufficiently with frequent water changes, about ten percent of the carbohydrates will dissolve into solution. Keep in mind that when bacon is cooked to a moderate temperature, nearly half of its fat content is lost.

There are several rather tasty breads that can be prepared for people with diabetes, but most so-called "gluten" and "diabetic flours" are complete scams, frequently containing as much as fifty or sixty percent. carbohydrates. It should be kept in mind that any gluten flour, even if it only has a small amount of carbohydrates, should be used with caution if significant protein restriction is desired. Gluten flour is made by washing away the starch from wheat flour, leaving a residue that is rich in the vegetable protein gluten. The 1913 Connecticut Agricultural Experiment Station study, Part I, Section 1, "Diabetic Foods," provides a very useful overview of food product analysis for people with diabetes. While soy meal, casoid flour, Lyster's flour, "akoll" biscuits, and "proto-puffs" have been proven to have some utility, their high protein content typically makes it difficult to provide a severe diabetic with substantial amounts of these foods over an extended period of time. We know the flours listed below to be trustworthy.

Below are some recipes that we think you'll find helpful. The purpose of bran is to add weight, dilute the protein, and coincidentally help prevent or treat constipation.

Lyster And Bran Flour Muffins

- Two teaspoons of level fat
- two eggs
- Four teaspoons of 40% fat heavy cream
- Two cups of cleaned bran
- One box of Lyster flour
- Half a cup or less of water

Put cheesecloth over dried bran and let it soak for an hour. Change the water numerous times while washing by squeezing the water through and through. Pat dry.

Beat the eggs well after separating them. Melted fat, cream, and two beaten egg whites should be added to the egg yolks. Stir in the water, cleaned bran, and Lyster flour.

Turn out 18 muffins.

Food value total: 1049 calories, 2 grams of carbohydrates, 68 grams of fat, and 99 grams of protein.

5 grams of protein, 4 grams of fat, trace carbohydrates, and 58 calories make up one muffin.

Lyster Brothers, Andover, Massachusetts, created Lyster's Diabetic Flour.

Bran Dough

- Two cups of wheat bran
- Two tsp of melted butter
- two complete eggs
- One white egg

- Half a teaspoon of salt
- Half a grain of saccharine

After tying the bran with cheesecloth, let it soak for an hour. Squeeze water through and through to wash. Frequently change the water. Pat dry. Beat the saccharine with a half-teaspoon of water. Beat the eggs thoroughly. Stir together the bran, melted butter, beaten eggs, and saccharine. Beat the last of the egg white and fold it in last. Using a tablespoon and a knife, form into little cakes. Grease a baking sheet and bake till golden brown.

You can get about 25 little cakes out of this mixture. 16 calories are contained in one cake. After this recipe's sample cake was examined, it was discovered that it had no sugar or starch.

Bran Muffins And Soya MIlk

- 30 grams (1 ounce) of soy meal
- 15 grams (1 level tablespoon) of butter
- 30 c.c. (1 ounce) 40% cream
- One cup of cleaned bran (follow directions elsewhere)
- One white egg
- One egg white can be swapped out for one entire egg.
- 1/4 tsp salt
- one and a half tsp baking powder

Combine baking powder, salt, and soy meal. To the cleaned bran, add. Add the cream and melted butter. Fold beaten egg white into mixture. To make a very thick drop batter, add extra water. Bake for fifteen to twenty-five minutes, or until golden brown, in six muffin tins that have been thoroughly oiled.

Value of food overall:

- 11 grams of protein and 27 grams of fat.
- Two grams of carbs. Total calories: 304.
- One muffin has 4.5 grams of fat and 2 grams of protein.
- trace of carbohydrates. 50 calories.

Bran Muffins And Casoid Flour

- 30 grams (1 ounce) of casoid flour
- 15 grams (1 level tablespoon) of butter
- 30 c.c. (1 ounce) 40% cream
- One white egg
- One egg white can be swapped out for one entire egg.
- 1/4 tsp salt
- one and a half tsp baking powder
- One cup of clean bran

Technique similar to the preceding rule. Use six muffin tins to bake.

Value of food overall:

- Eighteen grams of protein. Twenty-four grams of fat.
- One gram of carbohydrates. 300 calories.
- Three grams of protein per muffin. Four grams of fat.
- 50 cal of carbs plus calories.

Bran Muffins And Lyster Flour

- 30 grams (1 ounce) of yeast flour
- 15 grams (1 level tablespoon) of butter
- 30 c.c. (1 ounce) 40% cream
- One white egg
- One egg white can be swapped out for one entire egg.
- one-eighth teaspoon of salt
- One tsp baking powder
- One cup of clean bran

Same procedure as in the earlier recipe. Use six muffin tins to bake.

Value of food overall:

- Eighteen grams of protein. Twenty-five grams of fat.
- One gram of carbohydrates. Three hundred and sixty calories.
- Three grams of protein per muffin. Four grams of fat.
- Trace of carbohydrates. 50 calories.

Some recipes for special foods suitable for diabetics are provided to prevent a diet becoming repetitive. The majority of these recipes can be incorporated into diets with moderate calorie values. They are from Fannie Merritt Farmer's "Food and Cookery for the Sick and Convalescent."

Note: One full egg may be used in place of one egg white in the three recipes that came before it. The final product will have a little better texture but a somewhat higher food value.

MANUALS

Eggs With Butter.

Transfer one tsp of butter to a small omelet dish. After melting the butter, crack one egg into a cup and place it into the pan. Season with salt and pepper, then cook, rotating once, until the white is firm. It is important to take care not to crack the yolk.

A Beurre Noir Eggs.

Transfer one tsp of butter to a small omelet dish. Pour one egg into a cup and place it into the pan as soon as the butter has melted. Season with salt and pepper, then cook, rotating once, until the white is firm. It is important to take care not to crack the yolk. Transfer to a warm serving plate. Melt half a tablespoon of butter in the same pan, simmer until browned, and then stir in 1/4 tsp vinegar. Cover the egg with liquid.

Egg × La Suisse.

Put a buttered muffin ring inside a small omelet pan that has been heated. Add 1/4 teaspoon of butter, then 1 tablespoon of cream once it has melted. Crack one egg into a cup, place it in a muffin ring, and heat until the whites are set. Then, take out the ring and gradually cover the egg with a teaspoon of cream until it is cooked through. When almost done, add a pinch of salt, pepper, and a half-teaspoon of shredded cheese. Transfer the egg to a warm serving dish and cover with the leftover cream from the pan.

Egg Dropped.

Grease a muffin tin, then place it over hot water in an iron skillet with a tablespoon and a half of salt added. Crack the egg into the saucer and slide it into the ring so that the water covers it. Cover and place behind the range. Wait until the egg white takes on the consistency of jelly. Using an oiled griddle-cake turner, pick up the ring and egg and place them on a serving plate. Take off the ring and add parsley to the egg.

Dropping Egg Containing Tomato Puree.

Serve one spoonful of tomato purée alongside a dropped egg. To make tomato purée, boil and drain the tomatoes, then let them reduce to a thick consistency. Season with a little vinegar, salt, and pepper. You can also add a grating of horseradish root.

Igg Farci.

Halve a single "hard boiled" egg lengthwise. After removing the yolk, run it through a sieve. Clean the liver of one half of the bird, chop it finely, and sauté it in just enough butter to keep it from browning. Add a few drops of onion juice while cooking. Add to egg yolk; season with 1/4 tsp finely chopped parsley, salt, and pepper. Pour mixture back into whites, top with grated cheese, and bake until cheese is melted. Accompany with a tsp of tomato purée.

Egg Farci Ii.

Prepare one egg as you would for Egg Farci I. Add to the yolk a half-ton of shredded cheese, a quarter-teaspoon of vinegar, a few grains of mustard, and salt and cayenne to taste. Finally, add enough melted butter to make the mixture the proper consistency for shaping. Refill whites and form into balls the size of the original yolks. Place in a pan of boiling water, cover, and leave to stand until fully heated. Arrange on a serving dish. Put a tiny bit of parsley into each yolk.

Baked Tomato Egg.

Scoop out the pulp from a medium-sized tomato by cutting a slice at the stem end. Place one egg into the created cavity, season with salt and pepper, cover, place in a small baking pan, and bake for the egg to set.

Egg Steamed.

Lightly coat each individual earthen mould with a thick layer of butter. One-fourth teaspoon salt and a few grains of pepper are used to season two tablespoons of chopped cooked chicken, veal, or lamb. Put some meat in a greased mold and then crack in one egg. Cook the egg in a moderate oven until it sets. Remove off the mold and sprinkle with parsley.

Soup With Chicken And Beef Extract.

Half a cup of chicken broth

Half a teaspoon of Sauterne

one-eighth teaspoon pure beef

one and a half tablespoons of cream

Add pepper and salt.

Bring the stock to a boil before adding the other ingredients.

Soup Of Chicken With Egg Custard.

Serve egg custard alongside chicken soup.

Egg Custard: Lightly beat the yolk of one egg, then whisk in a half-teaspoon each of cream and water, season with salt. Fill a tiny buttered tin mold, set it in a pan of hot water, and bake it until it solidifies. Once cooled, take it out of the mold and cut it into creative forms.

Soup With Chicken And Egg Balls I Or Ii.

Egg Balls I: Sift the yolk of one hard-boiled egg, add salt and pepper to taste, and then add enough raw egg yolk to achieve the desired consistency for shaping. Shape into little spheres and simmer in broth.

Egg Balls II: Grate half of the yolk from a hard-boiled egg and add it to a finely chopped half of the hard-boiled egg white. Sprinkle with salt and beat in raw egg yolk until the proper consistency is reached for shaping. Just like with Egg Balls I, form and poach.

Royal Custard With Chicken Souper.

Serve Royal Custard alongside Chicken Soup.

Royal Custard: Lightly beat the yolk of one egg, whisk in two tablespoons chicken stock, season with pepper and salt, pour into a tiny buttered mold, and bake in a hot water pan until set. Once cooled, take out of the mold and slice into adorable shapes or little cubes.

Soup With Onions.

Simmer half of a large onion, thinly sliced, for eight minutes in one tablespoon of butter. After adding 1/4 cup of chicken stock, simmer for

20 minutes. Pass through a strainer, then whisk in two tablespoons of cream and half of beaten egg yolk. Add pepper and salt for seasoning.

Asparagus Soup.

- twelve asparagus stems, or
- one-third cup of asparagus tips in cans
- two and a third cups chicken stock
- 1/4 of an onion slice.
- Just one yolk
- One spoonful of heavy cream
- one-eighth teaspoon of salt
- A small amount of granules pepper

Pour cold water over the asparagus, bring it to a boil, then drain and add the onion and stock. Simmer for eight minutes, then rub the asparagus through a sieve, reheat, and add the cream, egg, and seasonings. After straining, serve.

Bisque Tomato.

- 2.3 cups of canned tomatoes
- one-fourth of an onion slice
- A small piece of bay leaf
- two cloves
- 1/4 cup of water that is boiling
- one-eighth teaspoon of soda
- Half a spoonful of butter
- 1/4 tsp salt
- A small amount of granules pepper
- Two teaspoons of heavy cream

For eight minutes, cook the first five ingredients. Put through a sieve, then stir in the cream, soda, and small bits of butter and seasoning. Serve right away.

Cauliflower Soup.

- one-third cup prepared cauliflower
- two and a third cups chicken stock
- little celery stalks
- one-fourth of an onion slice
- One yolk from an egg
- One spoonful of heavy cream
- two tsp of butter
- Add pepper and salt.

Stalk of cauliflower, celery, and onion should cook for 8 minutes. Run through a purée sieve, warm, then stir in the cream, butter, spices, and a little beaten egg yolk.

Soup With Mushrooms.

- Three shimps
- two and a third cups chicken stock
- one-fourth of an onion slice
- two tsp of butter
- One yolk from an egg
- One spoonful of heavy cream
- One teaspoon of sauterne
- Add pepper and salt.

After cleaning, chop, and cook for five minutes with one teaspoon of butter. After adding the stock, simmer for 8 minutes. Pass through a purée strainer and mix in the wine, cream, leftover butter, spices, and a little beaten egg yolk.

Soup with Spinach.

- One tablespoon of chopped, boiled spinach
- two and a third cups chicken stock
- One yolk from an egg
- One spoonful of heavy cream
- Add pepper and salt.

Simmer spinach for eight minutes with stock. Pass through a purée sieve, warm, then stir in the cream, spices, and a little beaten egg yolk.

Cucumber sauce, broiled fish.

Present a petite portion of pan-fried halibut, salmon, or swordfish accompanied by cucumber sauce.

Cucumber Sauce: Peel, grate, and strain half of a cucumber. Add vinegar, salt, and pepper for seasoning.

Cooked haliputé fillet with Hollandaise sauce.

Clean a little halibut fillet and secure with a skewer. Place in pan, top with buttered paper, sprinkle with salt and pepper, and bake for twelve minutes. Accompany with

Hollandaise Sauce: In a small sauce pan, combine one egg yolk, one tablespoon butter, and one teaspoon lemon juice. Place the sauce pan inside a bigger one that is filled with water. Using a wooden spoon, stir the mixture continuously until the butter melts. Next, add a half-teaspoon of butter, and then another half-teaspoon as the mixture thickens; season with cayenne and salt. This sauce is nearly viscous enough to maintain its structure. This sauce can be varied by adding a third teaspoon of grated horseradish or one-eighth teaspoon of beef extract to the first mixture.

Halibut Baked With Tomato Sauce.

After giving a tiny slice of halibut a wipe, season with salt and pepper. Place in buttered pan, top with a thin slice of fat, salt pork that has been gashed multiple times, and bake for 12 to 15 minutes. When the fish is ready to be served, remove the pork. Simmer one-third cup tomatoes, one clove, one-fourth onion slice, and a few grains with salt and pepper for eight minutes. Run through a strainer after removing the onion and clove. Simmer the tomato until it reduces to two tablespoons after adding a few grains of soda. Drizzle over fish and sprinkle with parsley.

Cheese With Halibut.

Season a tiny halibut fillet with salt and pepper, cover with melted butter, put it in the oven, and bake it for twelve minutes. Transfer to a serving platter and cover with the sauce of your choice:

Heat two teaspoons of cream, then beat in half of an egg yolk until thoroughly combined. Finally, stir in one spoonful of shredded cheese. Add paprika and salt for seasoning.

Finnian Haddi À La Demonica.

Place a tiny piece of finnan haddie in cold water, cover it, and place it on the back of the range. Let the water heat up gradually until it reaches boiling point, then let it remain below it for twenty minutes. After completely draining and rinsing, divide into flakes; two teaspoons should result. Reheat one hard-boiled egg, thinly sliced, in two tablespoons heavy cream over hot water. Add a teaspoon of butter, little salt, paprika, and finely chopped parsley for garnish.

Haddock Fillet With Wine Sauce.

Take off the skin off a tiny piece of haddock, place it in a baking pan with butter on it, and cover it with one tablespoon of white wine, one teaspoon of melted butter, and a few drops of each of lemon and onion juice. Bake with a cover on. Transfer to a serving plate, then whisk in one tablespoon of cream and one barely beaten egg yolk to the wine in the pan. Add pepper and salt for seasoning. Pour the strainer over the fish and top with finely chopped parsley.

Cool Cream Sauce Smelts.

After cleaning two chosen smelts, make five diagonal incisions on each of their sides. Add lemon juice, salt, and pepper for seasoning. After five minutes, cover and leave. Coat in milk, shake in flour, and fry in butter. Transfer to a serving plate and add two tablespoons of cream to the fat in the pan. After three minutes of cooking, season with a little lemon juice, salt, and pepper. Pour sauce over smelts and top with parsley that has been finely chopped.

Smilt Is The Maître Of The Hotel.

Melts should be prepared similarly to smelts with cream and served with butter from the maître d'hotel.

Codfish Salted With Cream.

Two teaspoons of salt codfish should be picked into flakes. Once soft, cover with lukewarm water and leave on the back of the range. Once the cream is hot, add the yolk of one tiny egg that has been lightly beaten. Drain and then add three tablespoons of cream.

Codfish Salted With Cheese.

Add a half tablespoon of shredded cheese and a few grains of paprika to the salted codfish with milk.

Sauce FIGARO, BROILED BEEFSTEAK.

Present a slice of grilled steak paired with Figaro Sauce.

Sauce Figaro: Add one teaspoon of tomato purée to the Hollandaise sauce. Put the tomatoes through a strainer and simmer until they are reduced to a thick pulp to make tomato purée stew tomatoes.

Horseradish cream sauce and roast beef.

Present a rare roast beef slice accompanied with a Horseradish Cream Sauce.

Cream Sauce with Horseradish: Beat 1 tablespoon heavy cream until it stiffens. Add the three-quarters teaspoon of vinegar gradually as the cream starts to thicken. Add a pinch of salt and pepper for seasoning, and then mix in half a tablespoon of shredded horseradish root.

A Fully Filled Beef.

Remove any excess fat from a thick tenderloin slice. Place in a heated skillet with three tablespoons of butter. Turn, sear one side, then sear the other. Simmer for eight minutes, rotating the dish periodically, making sure the whole surface is charred to stop the juices from seeping out.

Transfer to a warm serving dish and cover with the fat in the pan that has been cheesecloth-strained. Add sautéed mushroom caps, reheated and seasoned canned string beans, and cooked cauliflower as garnish.

Chops Of Lamb, Fineste Sauce.

Serve the lamb chops with Fineste Sauce.

Sauce Fineste: Melt a tablespoon and a half of butter. Add two tablespoons of stewed and strained tomatoes, a quarter teaspoon of Worcestershire sauce, a few drops of lemon juice, and a few grains of each of mustard and cayenne.

Spinach.

Drain and chop 1 cup of cooked spinach as dry as possible. Add salt and pepper for seasoning, filter through a purée sieve, and reheat in butter, using as much as the spinach will allow. Place onto a platter and top with a slice of hard-boiled egg white and a strainer-driven yolk.

Sprouts Of Brussels With Curry Sauce.

Remove any wilted leaves from the Brussels sprouts and let them soak in cold, salted water for fifteen minutes. Simmer in hot, salted water for twenty minutes, or until a skewer can easily be inserted and removed. After draining, cover with 1/4 cup of curry sauce.

Curry Sauce: Combine 1/4 teaspoon mustard, 1/4 teaspoon salt, and a small pinch of paprika. Add one tablespoon olive oil, one and a half tablespoons vinegar, a few drops of onion juice, and the yolk of one egg that has been lightly beaten. Stirring continuously, cook over hot water until mixture thickens. Add one teaspoon of melted butter, one-eighth teaspoon of chopped parsley, and one-fourth teaspoon of curry powder.

Cauliflower Fried.

Boil or steam a tiny cauliflower. After cooling, divide into pieces. Heat up enough olive oil to sauté food for one serving. Sprinkle with salt and pepper, place on a serving platter, and drizzle with 1 tablespoon of melted butter.

Huntington À Cauliflower.

Cut the steaming cauliflower into pieces and serve it with the same curry sauce sauce that you used for the Brussels sprouts.

Hollandaise Sauce Dressed Cauliflower.

Serve baked halibut fillet with Hollandaise sauce and boiled cauliflower as directed.

Cream-colored mushrooms.

Peel, wash, and cut six medium-sized mushroom caps into pieces. Sauté for three minutes in half a tablespoon of butter. Add one and one-half tablespoons cream and cook until mushrooms are tender. Season with salt and pepper and a slight grating of nutmeg.

Broiled Mushrooms.

Clean mushrooms, remove stems, and place caps on a buttered broiler. Broil five minutes, having gills nearest flame during first half of broiling. Arrange on serving dish, put a small piece of butter in each cap and sprinkle with salt and pepper.

Supreme Of Chicken.

Force breast of uncooked chicken through a meat chopper; there should be one-fourth cup. Add one egg beaten slightly and one-fourth cup heavy cream. Add pepper and salt for seasoning. Turn into slightly buttered mould, set in pan of hot water and bake until firm.

Sardine Relish.

Melt one tablespoon butter, and add two tablespoons cream. Heat to boiling point, add three sardines freed from skin and bones, and separated in small pieces, and one hard-boiled egg finely chopped. Season with salt and cayenne.

Diabetic Rarebit.

Beat two eggs slightly and add one-fourth teaspoon salt, a few grains cayenne, and two tablespoons, each, cream and water. Cook same as scrambled eggs, and just before serving add one-fourth Neufchâtel cheese mashed with fork.

Cheese Sandwiches.

Cream one-third tablespoon butter and add one-half tablespoon, each, finely chopped cold boiled ham and cold boiled chicken; then season with salt and paprika. Spread between slices of Gruyère cheese cut as thin as possible.

Cheese Custard.

Beat one egg slightly, add one-fourth cup cold water, two teaspoons heavy cream, one tablespoon melted butter, one tablespoon shredded cheese and a few grains salt. Turn into an individual mould, lay in pan of boiling water, and bake until firm.

Cold Slaw.

Select a small hefty cabbage, remove outside leaves, and cut cabbage in quarters; with a sharp knife slice extremely thinly. Soak in cold water until crisp; drain, dry between towels, and blend with cream salad dressing.

Cabbage Salad.

Finely shred one-fourth of a small crisp cabbage. Let stand two hours in salted cold water, allowing one tablespoon of salt to a pint of water. Cook slowly thirty minutes one-fourth cup, each, vinegar and cold water, with a touch of bay leaf, one-fourth teaspoon peppercorns, one-eighth teaspoon mustard seed and three cloves. Strain and pour over cabbage drained from salted water. Let stand two hours, again drain, and serve with or without mayonnaise dressing.

Cabbage And Celery Salad.

Wash and scrape two stalks of celery, add an equal number of shredded cabbage, and six walnut meats broken in pieces. Serve with cream dressing.

Cucumber Cup.

Pare a cucumber and cut in quarters cross wise. Remove center from one piece and fill cup thus prepared with tartare sauce. Present on a leaf of lettuce.

Cucumber And Leek Salad.

Cut cucumber in little cubes and leeks in extremely thin slices. Mix, using equal portions, and serve with French dressing.

Salad with cucumber and watercress.

Slice the cucumbers very thinly, then score the edges of each slice with a three-tined fork. Place atop a watercress bed.

Eggsalad I.

One hard-boiled egg should be cut in half crosswise so that the tops of the halves may remain pointed. Take out the yolk, mash it, add some cream or mayonnaise dressing to moisten it, form it into balls, add more egg whites, and serve it on lettuce leaves. Add a radish slice that is thin enough to resemble a tulip as a garnish.

Eggsalad.

The egg should be prepared similarly to Egg Salad I, with an equal amount of chopped cooked chicken or veal added to the yolk.

Cheese And Egg Salad.

The same steps as for Egg Salad I should be followed to prepare the egg. Add three-fourths of a spoonful of shredded cheese to the yolk, season with salt, pepper, and a few mustard grains, and then moisten with melted butter and vinegar. Dress salad or serve it plain.

Salad With Egg And Cucumber.

Slice thinly one hard-boiled egg. Cut a cooled cucumber into as many thin slices as there are egg pieces. Place in a circle shape, with the cucumber and egg slices overlapping one another. Use watercress or chicory to fill up the center. Accompany with a salad dressing.

Cheese Salad.

Half a Neufchâtel cheese should be mashed and then moistened with cream. Form into shapes that resemble robin eggs. Place on a lettuce leaf and top with dried parsley that has been chopped finely. Accompany with a salad dressing.

Oleive Salad With Cheese.

After mashing one-eighth of a cream cheese, add cayenne and salt to taste. Add two finely chopped lettuce leaves, some finely chopped olives, and a tiny bit of canned pimento to add some color. Press the cheese into its original shape, then leave it for two hours. Slice, then arrange on lettuce leaves with mayonnaise dressing on the side.

Cheese Salad With Tomatoes.

One medium-sized tomato should be peeled, chilled, and a small amount of pulp should be removed. Equal amounts of Neufchâtel and

Roquefort cheese should be combined, mashed, and then moistened with French dressing. Stuff cheese into the tomato hole. Serve with French dressing on top of lettuce leaves.

First fish salad.

Take the salmon out of the can, give it a good rinse in hot water, then cut it into pieces; there should be around 1/4 cup. Combine 1/8 teaspoon salt, a few grains of mustard and paprika, 1 teaspoon melted butter, 1/2 tablespoon cream, 1 tablespoon water, 1/2 tablespoon vinegar, and the yolk of 1 egg. Heat the mixture over hot water until it thickens, and then stir in 1/4 teaspoon granulated gelatin soaked in 1 teaspoon cold water. Mix into salmon, shape, refrigerate, and present with cucumber sauce.

Cucumber Sauce: Quarter a cucumber, cut, strain, and taste-test with French dressing.

Salad ASPARAGUS.

Four canned asparagus stalks should be drained and rinsed. Chop off a third of an inch wide ring from the red pepper. Arrange the asparagus stalks on top of the lettuce leaves, insert the ring, and drizzle with the French dressing.

Jelly Tomato Salad.

Add one-third teaspoon of granulated gelatin that has been soaked in a teaspoon of cold water to one-fourth cup of hot, stewed, and strained tomato. Pour into a single mold, freeze, remove from mold, place on top of lettuce leaves, and top with mayonnaise dressing.

Frozen Salad Of Tatsou.

Add a little cayenne and salt to the strained and cooked tomato. Pour mixture into tiny tin box, cover with buttered paper, insert tight fitting cover, add equal parts salt and ice, and leave for two hours. Take it out of the mold, put it on a lettuce leaf, and serve it with mayo.

Kale salad with tomatoes and vegetables.

Cook one-third cup of tomatoes for eight minutes along with a clove, four peppercorns, a sprig of parsley, and a sixth slice of onion. Take out the veggies and strain the tomato through a strainer; about 1/4 cup should come out. Add four drops vinegar, a few grains of salt, and one-eighth teaspoon of granulated gelatin steeped in one teaspoon of cold water. Pour mixture into individual mold; line with cucumber slices cut into interesting shapes and string beans. After chilling, take out of the mold, place on a lettuce leaf, and top with mayonnaise dressing.

A Bounty Of Tomatoes.

Slice a medium-sized tomato, leaving the stem end on top of the handle, into the shape of a basket. Put two halves of English walnut meats, chopped into small pieces and coated with French dressing, into the basket along with some cold cooked string beans. Present on a leaf of lettuce.

Salad With Tomato And Chive.

Take off the little tomato's skin. Chill and slice in half lengthwise. Drizzle with mayonnaise, top with finely chopped chives, and present on a leaf of lettuce.

Salad Canary.

Taking a slice off the stem end of a vibrant red apple, remove as much pulp as possible while preserving the contour of the shell. Using twice as much grapefruit as celery, fill shell created this way with grapefruit pulp and finely chopped celery. It will be required to remove a portion of the grapefruit's juice. Apply mayonnaise dressing, put the cover back on, and place on a lettuce leaf. Garnish with a canary made of Neufchâtel cheese, which has been shaped and colored yellow, has paprika eyes, and has a few grains on its body. Add three cheese eggs that are sprinkled with paprika and tinted green as garnish as well.

Note: Avoid using apple pulp.

Classical Salad.

Slice a chosen lemon into the shape of a handle-equipped basket, then remove all of the pulp. Place one tablespoon of cold, cooked chicken or sweet bread, cut into small dice, in the basket. Combine it with half a tablespoon of small cucumber dice and one teaspoon of finely chopped celery that has been wet with mayonnaise or cream dressing. Drizzle with dressing and garnish with thin slices of finely chopped round red radishes. Place a tiny parsley sprig on top of the handle. Place atop watercress.

Boats Cucumber.

Slice a little cucumber lengthwise in half. Remove the center and cut the shape of a boat. Dice the cucumber from the boats into small pieces, then finely chop one and a half olives. Drizzle with French dressing, transfer mixture into boats, and arrange on top of lettuce leaves.

Salad Of Spinach.

1/4 cup cooked spinach should be drained and chopped finely. Add melted butter, lemon juice, salt, and pepper for seasoning. Firmly fill each individual mold, cool, take out of mold, and place on a thin, circular-sliced piece of cooked tongue. Top with tartare sauce and garnish with a parsley wreath on the mold base.

Tartare Sauce: Add equal amounts of finely chopped capers, pickles, olives, and parsley to one tablespoon of mayonnaise dressing.

Cucumber Salad With Sweetbread.

Combine one tablespoon of cubed cucumber, two pieces of cold-cooked sweetbread, and half a tablespoon of finely chopped celery. After adding one-eighth teaspoon of granulated gelatin dissolved in one teaspoon of hot water and three-fourths teaspoon of vinegar, beat one and a half tablespoons of heavy cream until stiff. Place in a pan of icy water, then add the veggies and sweetbreads as the stew starts to thicken. Chill and mould. Take out of the mold, place on lettuce leaves, and add a cucumber slice and parsley sprig on the top.

Nut And Chicken Salad.

Combine two tablespoons of chilled, cooked chicken or turkey cubes with one tablespoon of finely chopped celery and half a tablespoon of oven-browned English walnut meats mixed with one-eighth teaspoon butter, a pinch of salt, and several grains of kosher salt before breaking into pieces. Apply mayonnaise dressing to dampen. Place coiled celery, celery tips, and entire nut meats on top of the mound as garnish.

Princess Pudding

- One yolk from an egg
- 3/4 tsp dissolved granulated gelatin in
- One tablespoon of water that has been brought to a boil
- two tsp lemon juice
- 1/4 teaspoon of dissolved saccharine
- one-fourth teaspoon of cold water
- one white egg.

Egg yolk should be thick and lemon-colored. Add gelatin and beat some more. Add the saccharine and lemon juice gradually as the mixture thickens. Fold in egg white, beaten until dry and stiff. Form a mold and set aside.

Bavaria Cream Coffee.

- two tsp coffee infusion
- One tablespoon of water
- Two teaspoons of heavy cream
- One yolk from an egg
- A small amount of salt granules
- One-third tsp finely ground gelatin dipped in
- 1 teaspoon cold water.
- One grain of sugar dissolved in
- half a teaspoon of cold water
- One white egg
- one-fourth teaspoon vanilla

Hot coffee, half a cream, and water. Once the mixture thickens, add the egg yolk that has been gently beaten. Next, add the salt and gelatin. Take off the heat source, allow it to cool down, then mix in the saccharine, stiffened cream, stiffened egg white, and a teaspoon of vanilla. Form a mold and refrigerate.

Sherbet with Lemon Cream.

- one-fourth cup cream
- two tsp cold water
- 1/2 teaspoon of dissolved saccharine
- half a teaspoon of cold water
- four lemon juice droplets
- A small amount of salt granules
- Place ingredients in the specified order and freeze.

Orange Ice.

- one-third cup of orange juice
- one tsp lemon juice
- two tsp cold water
- 1/2 teaspoon of dissolved saccharine
- half a teaspoon of cold water
- Combine ingredients in the specified order, then freeze.

Grapefruit Ice.

- 1/4 cup of grapefruit juice
- one-fourth cup water
- 1/2 teaspoon of dissolved saccharine
- half a teaspoon of cold water.

Extract grapefruit juice, drain, add additional ingredients, and freeze until smooth. Present in grapefruit parts.

Frosty Dish.

- one-fourth cup cream
- two tsp cold water
- one and a half teaspoons rum
- One yolk from an egg
- 1/2 teaspoon of dissolved saccharine
- half a teaspoon of cold water
- A small amount of salt granules

Add the egg yolk, which has been lightly beaten, and boil over hot water until the mixture thickens. Scald half of the cream with water. Add the other ingredients, cool, and then freeze.

MENU LISTS.

It is brought to light that the following diets have a relatively low protein allowance. The first two tables show the fast days; the remaining six show the transitional days, when food is progressively added but still falls short of the required number of calories. The remaining may be chosen based on the patient's weight or the case requirements.

One meat or one "5%" vegetable might be swapped out for another to add variation or avoid boredom. If more calories are required to maintain body weight, butter or olive oil can be added to the dish to boost the fat content. On the other hand, adding so much fat that the weight increases is not regarded as ideal.

TABLES

TABLE I.

Protein, 10 grams

Carbohydrate, 15 grams

Fat, 7 grams

Calories, 200

Breakfast.

String beans (canned).	120 grams	2-1/2 h. tbsp.
Asparagus (canned).	150 grams	3 h. tbsp. or 13-1/2 stalks 4 in. long.

Tea or coffee.

Dinner.

Celery.	100 grams	6 pieces 4-1/2 in. long.
Spinach (cooked).	135 grams	3 h. tbsp.

Tea or coffee.

Supper.

Asparagus.	100 grams	2 h. tbsp. or 9 stalks 4 in. long.
Celery.	100 grams	6 pieces 4-1/2 in. long.
Tea or coffee.		

TABLE II.

Protein, 7 grams

Carbohydrate, 15 grams

Fat, 6 grams

Calories, 150

Breakfast.

Asparagus (canned).	75 grams	1-3/4 h. tbsp. (chopped).
Cabbage.	65 grams	1 very h. tbsp.
Tea or coffee.		

Dinner.

Onions (cooked).	100 grams	2 h. tbsp.
Celery.	50 grams	3 pieces about 4-1/2 in. long.
Tea or coffee.		

Spinach.	100 grams	2 h. tbsp.
Celery.	50 grams	3 pieces 4-1/2 in. long.
Tea or coffee.		

TABLE III.

Protein, 24 grams

Carbohydrate, 8 grams

Fat, 22 grams

Calories, 340

BREAKFAST.

String beans.	100 grams	2 h. tbsp.
Egg.	1	
Coffee.		

DINNER.

Egg.	1	
Turnips.	100 grams	2 h. tbsp.
Cabbage.	100 grams	2 h. tbsp.
Tea.		

Egg.	1	
Turnips.	100 grams	2 h. tbsp.
Spinach.	100 grams	2 h. tbsp.
Tea.		

TABLE IV.

Protein, 31 grams

Fat, 14 grams

Carbohydrate, 17 grams

Calories, 327

BREAKFAST.

Egg.	1	
Asparagus.	100 grams	2 h. tbsp.
Tomatoes.	100 grams	2 h. tbsp.
Coffee.		

DINNER.

| Chicken. | 35 grams | 1 small serving. |
| String beans. | 200 grams | 4 h. tbsp. |

Cabbage.   100 grams   2 h. tbsp.

Tea or coffee.

SUPPER.

Egg.   1

Cauliflower.   240 grams   5 h. tbsp. +

Spinach.   100 grams   2 h. tbsp.

Tea or coffee.

TABLE V.

Protein, 43 grams

Carbohydrate,   15 grams

Fat, 19 grams

Calories, 414

BREAKFAST.

Egg.   1

Asparagus.   200 grams   4 h. tbsp.

Coffee.

DINNER.

Chicken.	70 grams	1 mod. serving.
Cauliflower.	120 grams	2 h. tbsp.
Cabbage (cooked).	100 grams	2 h. tbsp.
Tea.		

SUPPER.

Egg.	1	
String beans.	100 grams	2 h. tbsp.
Spinach.	200 grams	4 h. tbsp.
Tea.		

TABLE VI.

Protein, 38 grams

Fat, 31 grams

Carbohydrate, 19 grams

Calories, 520

BREAKFAST.

Egg.	1	
Asparagus.	200 grams	4 h. tbsp.
Coffee.		

DINNER.

Steak.	100 grams	1 small serving.
Celery (cooked).	200 grams	4 h. tbsp.
Tea.		

SUPPER.

Egg.	1	
Lettuce.	20 grams	2 medium leaves.
Cucumbers.	100 grams	2 h. tbsp.
String beans.	50 grams	1 h. tbsp.
Tea.		

TABLE VII.

Protein, 35 grams

Carbohydrate, 17 grams

Fat, 100 grams

Calories, 1143

BREAKFAST.

Bacon.	50 grams	2 slices about 6 in. long.

Asparagus.	100 grams	2 h. tbsp. or 9 stalks 4 in. long (canned).
Spinach.	100 grams	2 h. tbsp.
Butter.		
Cream.		
Coffee.		

DINNER.

Steak.	100 grams	1 small serving.
Turnips.	140 grams	2 h. tbsp. +
Spinach.	100 grams	2 h. tbsp.
Cabbage.	100 grams	2 h. tbsp.
Butter.		
Tea.		
Cream.		

SUPPER.

Spinach.	100 grams	2 h. tbsp.
String beans (cooked).	100 grams	2 h. tbsp.
Cauliflower (cooked).	120 grams	2 h. tbsp. +

Butter.

Tea.

Cream.

Allow during day:

Butter.	20 grams	2 squares.
Cream, 40%.	2-1/2 ounces	5 tbsp.

TABLE VIII.

Protein, 40 grams

Carbohydrate, 16 grams

Fat, 104 grams

Calories, 1196

BREAKFAST.

Egg.	1	
Asparagus.	100 grams	2 h. tbsp or 9 stalks 4 in. long (canned).
Spinach.	100 grams	2 h. tbsp.
Butter.		
Coffee.		

Cream.

DINNER.

Steak.	100 grams	1 small serving.
Turnips.	140 grams	2 h. tbsp. +
Celery.	100 grams	2 h. tbsp.
Cabbage.	100 grams	2 h. tbsp.
Butter.		
Cream.		
Tea.		

SUPPER.

Bacon.	50 grams	2 slices about 6 in. long.
Spinach.	100 grams	2 h. tbsp.
String beans (canned).	100 grams	2 h. tbsp.
Cauliflower.	100 grams	2 h. tbsp.
Butter.		
Cream.		
Tea.		

Allow during day:

| Butter. | 20 grams | 2 squares. |
| Cream 40%. | 3 ounces | 6 tbsp. |

TABLE IX.

Protein, 50 grams

Carbohydrate, 15 grams

Fat, 125 grams

Calories, 1500

BREAKFAST.

Eggs.	2	
String beans(canned).	100 grams	3 h. tbsp.
Butter.		
Cream.		
Coffee.		

DINNER.

Chop.	100 grams	1 chop.
Cabbage (cooked).	100 grams	2 h. tbsp.
Cucumbers.	100 grams	2 h. tbsp.
Tea.		

Butter.

Cream.

SUPPER.

Egg.	1	
Asparagus (canned).	100 grams	2 h. tbsp.
Cauliflower (cooked).	100 grams	2 h. tbsp.
Butter.		
Cream.		
Tea.		

Allow during day:

| Butter. | 25 grams | 2-1/2 square. |
| Cream, 40%. | 5 ounces | 10 tbsp. |

TABLE X.

Protein, 61 grams

Carbohydrate, 16 grams

Fat, 160 grams

Calories, 1795

BREAKFAST.

Bacon.	50 grams	2 slices 6 in. long.
Eggs.	2	
Spinach.	100 grams	2 h. tbsp.
Butter.		
Cream.		
Coffee.		

DINNER.

Steak.	100 grams	1 small serving.
Tomatoes (canned).	100 grams	2 h. tbsp.
Butter.		
Cream.		
Tea.		

SUPPER.

Chicken.	50 grams	1 small serving.
Lettuce.	20 grams	2 leaves.
Celery.	100 grams	6 stalks 4-1/2 in. long.

Butter.

Cream.

Tea.

Allow during day:

Butter.	50 grams	5 squares.
Cream, 40%.	5 ounces	10 tbsp.

TABLE XI.

Protein, 38 grams

Carbohydrate, 20 grams

Fat, 100 grams

Calories, 1168

BREAKFAST.

Bacon.	30 grams	1-1/2 slices 6 in. long.
Egg.	1	
Spinach.	100 grams	2 h. tbsp.
Coffee.		
Butter.		
Cream.		

DINNER.

Steak.	50 grams	1 very small serving.
Cabbage.	100 grams	2 h. tbsp.
Onions.	100 grams	2 h. tbsp.
Butter.		
Cream.		
Tea.		

SUPPER.

Scraped beef balls.	40 grams = 1-1/3 oz.	
Chopped celery salad.	100 grams	2 h. tbsp.
Tomatoes.	100 grams	2 tbsp.

Allow during day:

| Butter. | 25 grams | 2-1/2 squares. |
| Cream, 40%. | 4 ounces | 8 tbsp. |

TABLE XII.

Protein, 35 grams

Carbohydrate, 16 grams

Fat, 92 grams

Calories, 1064

Breakfast.

Egg.	1	
Cabbage.	100 grams	2 h. tbsp.
Tomatoes.	100 grams	2 h. tbsp.
Butter.		
Coffee.		
Cream.		

Dinner.

Steak.	80 grams	1 small serving.
Spinach.	100 grams	2 h. tbsp.
Turnips.	140 grams	2 h. tbsp. +
Egg, white.	1	
Butter.		
Cream.		
Tea.		

Supper.

Cauliflower.	120 grams	2 h. tbsp. +

Onions.	100 grams	2 h. tbsp.
Lettuce.	10 grams	1 leaf.
Olive oil.	5 grams	1 teaspoon. +
Tea.		
Butter.		
Cream.		

Allow during day:

| Butter. | 25 grams | 2-1/2 squares. |
| Cream, 40%. | 3 ounces | 6 tbsp. |

TABLE XIII.

Protein, 40 grams

Fat, 110 grams

Carbohydrate, 21 grams

Calories, 1187

BREAKFAST.

Bacon.	50 grams	2 slices 6 in. long.
Cauliflower.	120 grams	2 h. tbsp.
Butter.		

Cream.

Coffee.

DINNER.

Squab.	1	
Carrots.	100 grams	2 h. tbsp.
Tomatoes.	100 grams	2 h. tbsp.
Butter.		
Cream.		
Tea.		

SUPPER.

Turnips.	140 grams	2 h. tbsp. +
Asparagus.	100 grams	2 h. tbsp.
Celery.	100 grams	6 stalks 4-1/2 in. long.
Butter.		
Cream.		
Tea.		

Allow during day:

Butter.	20 grams	2 squares.
Cream, 40%.	3-1/2 ounces	7 tbsp.

<h1 style="text-align:center">TABLE XIV.</h1>

Protein, 40 grams

Carbohydrate,   20 grams

Fat, 103 grams

Calories, 1200

Breakfast.

Egg.	1 + 1 egg white.	
Spinach.	200 grams	4 h. tbsp.
Cream.		
Butter.		

Dinner.

Steak.	50 grams	1 very small serving.
Cabbage.	100 grams	2 h. tbsp.
Tomatoes.	100 grams	2 h. tbsp.
Onions.	100 grams	2 h. tbsp.
Butter.		
Cream.		

Tea.

Supper.

Scraped beef balls	40 grams	1-1/3 oz.
Celery.	100 grams	6 stalks 4-1/2 in. long.
Cream.		
Butter.		
Tea.		

Allow during day:

| Butter. | 20 grams | 2 squares. |
| Cream, 40%. | 5 ounces | 10 tbsp. |

TABLE XV.

Protein, 40 grams

Carbohydrate,   22 grams

Fat, 105 grams

Calories, 2100

Breakfast.

| Egg. | 1 | |
| Asparagus. | 100 grams | 2 h. tbsp. |

Butter.

Cream.

Coffee.

DINNER.

Chop.	105 grams	1 medium.
Peas.	50 grams	1 h. tbsp.
Celery.	50 grams	6 stalks 4-1/2 in. long.

Butter.

Cream.

Tea.

SUPPER.

Cauliflower.	120 grams	2 h. tbsp. +
String beans.	100 grams	2 h. tbsp.

Butter.

Cream.

Tea.

Allow during day:

Butter.	20 grams	2 squares.
Cream, 40%.	4 ounces	8 tbsp.

TABLE XVI.

Protein, 40 grams

Fat, 100 grams

Carbohydrate, 30 grams

Calories, 1200

B̲REAKFAST.

Bacon.	50 grams	2 slices 6 in. long.
Peas (canned).	75 grams	1-3/4 h. tbsp.
Butter.		
Cream.		
Coffee.		

D̲INNER.

Broth—6 ounces with vegetables:

Cabbage.	25 grams	1 level tbsp.
Tomatoes.	25 grams	1 level tbsp.
Turnips.	25 grams	1 level tbsp.
Celery.	50 grams	3 pieces 4-1/2 in. long.

Steak.	100 grams	1 small serving.
Squash.	50 grams	1 h. tbsp.
Tomatoes.	75 grams	1-3/4 tbsp.
Butter.		
Cream.		
Tea.		

Supper.

Spinach.	100 grams	2 h. tbsp.
Turnips.	175 grams	3-3/4 h. tbsp.
Celery.	100 grams	6 stalks 4-1/2 in. long.

Allow during day:

| Butter. | 50 grams | 5 squares. |
| Cream, 40%. | 4 ounces | 8 tbsp. |

TABLE XVII.

Protein, 40 grams

Carbohydrate, 30 grams

Fat, 100 grams

Calories, 1200

Breakfast.

Bacon.	50 grams	2 slices about 6 in. long.
Egg.	1	
Asparagus (chopped).	100 grams	2 h. tbsp.
Butter.		
Cream.		
Coffee.		

Dinner.

Chicken.	50 grams	1 small serving.
Cabbage.	100 grams	2 h. tbsp.
Cauliflower.	120 grams	2 h. tbsp. +
Cucumbers.	100 grams	2 h. tbsp.
Butter.		
Cream.		
Tea.		

Supper.

Turnips.	140 grams	2 h. tbsp.

String beans.	100 grams	2 h. tbsp.
Bread.	25 grams	1 thin slice, baker's loaf.
Butter.		
Cream.		
Tea.		

Allow during day:

| Butter. | 25 grams | 2-1/2 squares. |
| Cream, 40%. | 4 ounces | 8 tbsp. |

TABLE XVIII.

Protein, 40 grams

Carbohydrate, 35 grams

Fat, 110 grams

Calories, 1330

BREAKFAST.

Bacon.	50 grams	2 slices about 6 in. long.
Peas.	75 grams	1-3/4 h. tbsp.
Tomatoes.	100 grams	2 h. tbsp.

Butter.

Cream.

Coffee.

Dinner.

Broth—chicken, lamb or beef.	6 ounces	
Steak.	100 grams	1 small serving.
Turnips.	200 grams	4 h. tbsp.
Celery.	150 grams	9 stalks 4-1/2 in. long.
Butter.		
Cream.		
Tea.		

Supper.

Squash.	50 grams	1 h. tbsp.
Beets.	100 grams	2 h. tbsp.
Cabbage (raw).	25 grams	1 h. tbsp.
Butter.		
Cream.		
Tea.		

Allow during day:

| Butter. | 25 grams | 2-1/2 squares. |
| Cream, 40%. | 4 ounces | 8 tbsp. |

TABLE XIX.

Protein, 40 grams

Carbohydrate, 35 grams

Fat, 115 grams

Calories, 1370

BREAKFAST.

Bacon.	50 grams	3 slices 6 in. long.
Parsnips.	100 grams	2 h. tbsp.
Potatoes (boiled).	50 grams	1 very small one.
Butter.		
Cream.		
Coffee.		

DINNER.

| Broth. | 6 ounces | |

Squab.	1	
Cabbage.	100 grams	2 h. tbsp.
Celery.	100 grams	6 stalks about 4-1/2 in. long.
Butter.		
Cream.		
Tea.		

SUPPER.

String beans.	140 grams	3 h. tbsp.
Cucumbers.	100 grams	2 h. tbsp.
Parsnips.	100 grams	2 h. tbsp.
Cauliflower.	120 grams	2 h. tbsp. +
Milk.	4 ounces	1/2 glass.
Butter.		
Cream.		
Tea.		

Allow during day:

Butter.	20 grams	2 squares.
Cream, 40%.	4 ounces	8 tbsp.

TABLE XX.

Protein, 50 grams

Carbohydrate, 35 grams

Fat, 130 grams

Calories, 1557

Breakfast.

Orange.	100 grams	1 small.
Bacon.	50 grams	3 slices, 6 in. long.
Egg.	1	
Spinach.	100 grams	2 h. tbsp.
Butter.		
Cream.		
Coffee.		

Dinner.

Broth.	180 c.c.	1 glass or cup.
Steak.	100 grams	1 small serving.
Boiled onions.	100 grams	2 h. tbsp.
Butter.		

Cream.

Tea.

Supper.

Egg.	1	
Lettuce.	25 grams	3 small leaves.
Bread.	20 grams	1 very thin slice.
Cream.		
Tea.		
Butter.		

Allow during day:

Butter.	25 grams	2-1/2 squares.
Cream, 40%.	4 ounces	8 tbsp.

TABLE XXI.

Protein, 50 grams

Carbohydrate, 40 grams

Fat, 158 grams

Calories, 1830

Breakfast.

Bacon.	50 grams	2 slices 6 in. long.
Bread.	20 grams	1 slice, 3 x 3 x 1/2 in.
Spinach.	100 grams	2 h. tbsp.
Butter.		
Cream.		
Coffee.		

DINNER.

Broth.	180 c.c.	1 glass or cup.
Steak.	100 grams	1 small serving.
Cabbage.	100 grams	2 h. tbsp.
Lettuce.	100 grams	10 leaves.
Butter.		
Cream.		
Tea.		

SUPPER.

Egg.	1	
Onions (boiled).	100 grams	2 h. tbsp.

Bread.	15 grams	1 slice very thin, 3 x 3 x 1/4
Milk.	4 ounces	8 tbsp.
Butter.		
Cream.		
Tea.		

Allow during day:

Butter.	50 grams	5 squares.
Cream, 40%.	5 ounces	10 tbsp.

TABLE XXII.

Protein, 60 grams

Carbohydrate, 30 grams

Fat, 158 grams

Calories, 1830

BREAKFAST.

Bacon.	50 grams	2 slices 6 in. long.
Egg.	1	
Tomatoes.	100 grams	2 h. tbsp.

Cream.

Butter.

Coffee.

Dinner.

Steak.	100 grams	1 small serving.
Turnips.	420 grams	4 h. tbsp. +
Cucumbers.	100 grams	2 h. tbsp.
Onions.	100 grams	2 medium sized.

Butter.

Cream.

Tea.

Olive oil.	21 grams	1-1/2 tbsp.

Supper.

Chicken.	50 grams	1 small serving.
Lettuce.	100 grams	10 medium leaves.
Celery.	100 grams	6 stalks 4-1/2 in. long.
Spinach.	100 grams	2 h. tbsp.

Butter.

Tea.

Cream.

Allow during day:

| Butter. | 15 grams | 1-1/2 squares. |
| Cream, 40%. | 6 ounces | 12 tbsp. |

TABLE XXIII.

Protein, 62 grams

Carbohydrate, 31 grams

Fat, 153 grams

Calories, 1800

BREAKFAST.

Bacon.	50 grams	2 slices.
Peas.	75 grams	1-1/2 h. tbsp.
Butter.		
Cream.		
Coffee.		

DINNER.

Broth—100 c.c.   7 tbsp.
with vegetables: =

Cabbage.	25 grams	1 level tbsp.
Tomato.	25 grams	1 level tbsp.
Turnip.	25 grams	1 level tbsp.
Celery (chopped).	50 grams	2 level tbsp.
Steak.	100 grams	1 small serving.
Squash.	50 grams	1 h. tbsp.
Tomatoes.	75 grams	1-1/2 h. tbsp.
Butter.		
Cream.		
Tea.		

Supper.

Chicken.	75 grams	1 small serving.
Turnips.	175 grams	2-3/4 h. tbsp.
Celery.	100 grams	6 stalks 4-1/2 in. long.

Allow during day:

Butter.	50 grams	5 squares.

| Cream, 40%. | 5 ounces | 10 tbsp. |
| Olive oil. | 7 grams | 1/2 tbsp. + |

TABLE XXIV.

Protein, 60 grams

Carbohydrate, 30 grams

Fat, 158 grams

Calories, 1830

BREAKFAST.

Bacon.	50 grams	2 slices 6 in. long.
Egg.	1	
Turnips.	140 grams	3 h. tbsp. —
Butter.		
Cream.		
Coffee.		

DINNER.

| Steak. | 100 grams | 1 small serving. |
| Celery. | 100 grams | 6 stalks 4-1/2 in. long. |

Cucumbers.	100 grams	2 h. tbsp.
Lettuce.	100 grams	10 leaves.
Spinach.	100 grams	2 h. tbsp.
Olive oil.	21 grams	1-1/2 tbsp. +
Butter.		
Cream.		
Tea.		

SUPPER.

Chicken.	50 grams	1 very small serving.
Turnips.	280 grams	4 h. tbsp. +
Onions.	100 grams	2 h. tbsp.
Tomatoes.	100 grams	2 h. tbsp.
Butter.		
Cream.		
Tea.		

Allow during day:

| Butter. | 50 grams | 5 squares. |
| Cream, 40%. | 5 ounces | 10 tbsp. |

<h1 style="text-align:center">TABLE XXV.</h1>

Protein, 60 grams

Carbohydrate, 30 grams

Fat, 154 grams

Calories, 1800

BREAKFAST.

Bacon.	60 grams	2-1/2 slices, 6 in. long.
Eggs.	2	
Turnips.	140 grams	2-1/2 h. tbsp.

DINNER.

Steak.	100 grams	1 small serving.
Spinach.	50 grams	1 h. tbsp.
Parsnips.	150 grams	3 h. tbsp.
Onions.	100 grams	2 h. tbsp.
Beets.	50 grams	1 h. tbsp.
Butter.		
Cream.		
Tea.		

SUPPER.

Ham.	50 grams	1 very small serving.
Lettuce.	100 grams	10 leaves.
String beans.	50 grams	1 h. tbsp.
Celery.	100 grams	6 stalks 4-1/2 in. long.
Asparagus.	50 grams	1 h. tbsp.

Allow during day:

Butter.	40 grams	4 squares.
Cream, 40%.	4 ounces	8 tbsp.

TABLE XXVI.

Protein, 40 grams

Carbohydrate, 36 grams

Fat, 105 grams

Calories, 1280

BREAKFAST.

Bacon.	50 grams	2 slices.
Parsnips.	100 grams	2 h. tbsp.

Potatoes (mashed).	60 grams	1 h. tbsp.
Butter.		
Cream.		
Coffee.		

DINNER.

Broth.	180 c.c.	1 glass.
Squab.	100 grams	1 squab (small).
Cabbage.	100 grams	2 tbsp.
Celery.	100 grams	6 stalks 4-1/2 in. long.
Butter.		
Cream.		
Tea.		

SUPPER.

String beans.	100 grams	2 h. tbsp.
Cucumbers.	100 grams	2 h. tbsp.
Parsnips.	100 grams	2 h. tbsp.
Cauliflower.	120 c.c.	2 h. tbsp. +
Milk.	120 c.c.	1/2 glass.

Butter.

Cream.

Tea.

Allow during day:

Butter.	20 grams	2 squares.
Cream, 40%.	4 ounces	8 tbsp.

TABLE XXVII.

Protein, 50 grams

Carbohydrate, 40 grams

Fat, 131 grams

Calories, 1587

BREAKFAST.

Egg.	1	
Parsnips.	100 grams	2 h. tbsp.
Bread.	35 grams	1 slice, 3 x 3-1/2 x 1/2 in.

Butter.

Cream.

Coffee.

DINNER.

Broth.	180 c.c.	1 glass or cup.
Chop.	100 grams	1
Cauliflower.	120 grams	2 h. tbsp. +
Carrots.	100 grams	2 h. tbsp.
Butter.		
Cream.		
Tea.		

SUPPER.

Bacon.	50 grams	2 slices.
Lettuce.	25 grams	3 leaves.
String beans.	100 grams	2 h. tbsp.
Peas.	55 grams	1 h. tbsp. +
Spinach.	100 grams	2 h. tbsp.
Butter.		
Cream.		
Tea.		

Allow during day:

Butter.	25 grams	2-1/2 squares.

| Cream, 40%. | 3 ounces | 6 tbsp. |

TABLE XXVIII.

Protein, 50 grams

Carbohydrate, 50 grams

Fat, 124 grams

Calories, 1563

Breakfast.

Orange.	100 grams	1 small.
Eggs.	2	
Bread.	10 grams	1 slice, 2 x 1 x 1/2 in.
Butter.		
Cream.		
Coffee.		

Dinner.

Steak.	100 grams	1 small serving.
Lettuce.	100 grams	10 leaves.
Spinach.	100 grams	2 h. tbsp.

Butter.

Cream.

Tea.

Supper.

Egg.	1	
Cold ham.	50 grams	1 small serving.
Asparagus.	50 grams	1 h. tbsp.
String beans.	100 grams	2 h. tbsp.
Bread.	25 grams	1 slice, 3 x 3 x 1/2 in.

Butter.

Cream.

Tea.

Allow during day:

Butter.	30 grams	3 squares.
Cream, 40%.	4 ounces	8 tbsp.

TABLE XXIX.

Protein, 52 grams

Carbohydrate, 52 grams

Fat, 116 grams

Calories, 1504

BREAKFAST.

Orange.	100 grams	1 small.
Bacon.	50 grams	2 slices 6 in. long.
Egg.	1	
Bread.	20 grams	1 slice, 3 x 2 x 1/2 in.
Butter.		
Cream.		
Coffee.		

DINNER.

Boiled ham.	100 grams	1 large slice (thin).
Brussels sprouts.	100 grams	2 h. tbsp.
Milk.	6 ounces	1 glass.
Butter.		
Tea.		

Cream.

Supper.

Scotch broth.	6 ounces	12 tbsp.
Lettuce.	50 grams	5 leaves.
Bread.	20 grams	1 slice, 3 x 2 x 1/2 in.

Allow during day:

Butter.	20 grams	2 squares.
Cream, 40%.	3 ounces	6 tbsp.

TABLE XXX.

Protein, 50 grams

Carbohydrate, 50 grams

Fat, 117 grams

Calories, 1590

Breakfast.

Orange.	100 grams	1 small.
Bread.	25 grams	1 slice, 3 x 2 x 1/2 in.
Egg.	1	

Bacon.	50 grams	2 slices 6 in. long.
Butter.		
Cream.		
Coffee.		

DINNER.

Chop.	100 grams	1 medium chop.
Asparagus.	100 grams	2 h. tbsp.
Butter.		
Cream.		
Tea.		

SUPPER.

Egg.	1	
Cucumbers.	100 grams	2 h. tbsp.
Lettuce.	10 grams	1 leaf.
Bread.	25 grams	1 slice, 3 x 2 x 1/2 in.

Allow during day:

Butter.	30 grams	3 squares.
Cream, 40%.	3 ounces	6 tbsp.

TABLE XXXI.

Protein, 53 grams

Carbohydrate,   50 grams

Fat, 133 grams

Calories, 1658

BREAKFAST.

Orange.	150 grams	1 medium.
Bacon.	60 grams	2-1/2 slices.
Egg.	1	
Bread.	20 grams	1 slice, 3 x 2 x 1/2 in.
Butter.		
Cream.		
Tea.		

DINNER.

Steak.	50 grams	1 very small serving.
String beans.	50 grams	1 h. tbsp.
Lettuce.	100 grams	10 leaves.

Butter.

Cream.

Tea.

Supper.

Ham.	50 grams	1 small slice.
Asparagus.	50 grams	1 h. tbsp.
Spinach.	50 grams	1 h. tbsp.
Bread.	15 grams	1 slice, 3 x 1 x 1/2 in.

Butter.

Cream.

Tea.

Allow during day:

Butter.	20 grams	2 squares.
Cream, 40%.	3 ounces	6 tbsp.

TABLE XXXII.

Protein, 101 grams

Carbohydrate, 51 grams

Fat, 255 grams

Calories, 2995

Breakfast.

Orange.	50 grams	1/2 orange (small).
Steak.	100 grams	1 slice.
Egg.	1	
Bread.	20 grams	1 slice, 3 x 2 x 1/2 in.
Butter.		
Cream.		
Tea.		

Dinner.

Lamb chop.	180 grams	2 small.
Potato.	50 grams	1 very small.
Turnip.	140 grams	2 h. tbsp +
Lettuce.	10 grams	1 leaf.
Tomato (raw).	100 grams	1 medium.

Custard—made with one egg and part of the cream.

Butter.

Tea.

| Olive oil. | 1-1/2 tbsp. | |

SUPPER.

Bacon.	50 grams	2 slices 6 in. long.
Eggs.	2	
Onions.	50 grams	1 h. tbsp.
Cabbage.	100 grams	2 h. tbsp.
Bread.	20 grams	1 slice, 3 x 2 x 1/2 in.

Butter.

Cream.

Tea.

Allow during day:

| Butter. | 50 grams | 5 squares. |
| Cream, 40%. | 6 ounces | 12 tbsp. |

TABLE XXXIII.

Protein, 60 grams

Carbohydrate, 55 grams

Fat, 159 grams

Calories, 1950

BREAKFAST.

Orange.	100 grams	1 small.
Bacon.	100 grams	4 slices 6 in. long.
Egg.	1	
Spinach.	100 grams	2 h. tbsp.
Bread.	25 grams	1 slice, 3 x 2 x 1/2 in.
Butter.		
Cream.		
Coffee.		

DINNER.

Broth.	180 c.c.	1 glass or cup.
Steak.	100 grams	1 small serving.
Parsnips.	100 grams	2 h. tbsp.
Carrots.	100 grams	2 h. tbsp.
Butter.		
Cream.		

Tea.

Supper.

Egg.	1	
Lettuce.	25 grams	3 medium leaves.
String beans.	10 grams	2 h. tbsp.
Bread.	25 grams	1 slice, 3 x 2 x 1/2 in.
Spinach.	60 grams	1 very h. tbsp.
Butter.		
Cream.		
Tea.		

Allow during day:

Butter.	25 grams	2-1/2 squares.
Cream, 40%.	4 ounces	8 tbsp.

TABLE XXXIV.

Protein, 60 grams

Carbohydrate, 50 grams

Fat, 145 grams

Calories, 1800

Breakfast.

Egg.	1	
Bacon.	100 grams	4 slices 6 in. long.
Tomatoes.	100 grams	2 h. tbsp.
Bread.	35 grams	1 slice, medium.
Butter.		
Cream.		
Tea.		

Dinner.

Broth.	180 c.c.	1 glass or cup.
Squab.	100 grams	1 squab (small).
Cabbage.	100 grams	2 h. tbsp.
Onions.	100 grams	2 h. tbsp.
Butter.		
Cream.		
Tea.		

Supper.

Egg.	1	
Lettuce.	25 grams	3 medium leaves.
Celery.	100 grams	6 stalks, 4-1/2 in. long.
Bread.	30 grams	1 slice, med. thin.

Allow during day:

| Butter. | 30 grams | 3 squares. |
| Cream, 40%. | 3-1/2 ounces | 7 tbsp. |

TABLE XXXV.

Protein, 63 grams

Carbohydrate, 60 grams

Fat, 140 grams

Calories, 1800

BREAKFAST.

| Grape fruit. | 100 grams | 1/2 small grape fruit. |
| Bacon. | 100 grams | 4 slices 6 in. long. |

Egg.	1	
Cauliflower.	120 grams	2 h. tbsp. +
Bread.	30 grams	1 slice, med. thin.
Butter.		
Cream.		
Coffee.		

DINNER.

Broth.	180 c.c.	1 glass.
Squab.	100 grams	1 squab.
Carrots.	100 grams	2 h. tbsp.
Lettuce.	100 grams	10 leaves.
Asparagus.	100 grams	2 h. tbsp.
Butter.		
Cream.		
Tea.		

SUPPER.

Egg.	1	
Asparagus.	100 grams	2 h. tbsp.
Spinach.	100 grams	2 h. tbsp.

Bread.	30 grams	1 slice, med. thin.
Butter.		
Cream.		
Tea.		

Allow during day:

| Butter. | 20 grams | 2 squares. |
| Cream, 40%. | 3 ounces | 6 tbsp. |

TABLE XXXVI.

Protein, 60 grams

Carbohydrate, 60 grams

Fat, 140 grams

Calories, 1794

BREAKFAST.

Orange.	100 grams	1 small.
Bacon.	100 grams	4 slices 6 in. long.
Egg.	1	
Bread.	35 grams	1 slice medium.

Butter.

Cream.

Tea.

Dinner.

Broth.	180 c.c.	1 glass or cup.
Steak.	100 grams	1 small serving.
Turnips.	140 grams	2 h. tbsp. +
Parsnips.	200 grams	4 h. tbsp.
String beans.	100 grams	2 h. tbsp.

Butter.

Cream.

Tea.

Supper.

Egg.	1	
Lettuce.	25 grams	3 leaves.
Cucumbers.	100 grams	16 slices (thin).
Bread.	30 grams	1 slice, med. thin.

Butter.

Cream.

Tea.

Allow during day:

| Butter. | 20 grams | 2 squares. |
| Cream, 40%. | 3 ounces | 6 tbsp. |

TABLE XXXVII.

Protein, 74 grams

Carbohydrate, 62 grams

Fat, 179 grams

Calories, 2220

Breakfast.

Bacon.	100 grams	4 slices 6 in. long.
Egg.	1	
Bread.	30 grams	1 slice, 3 x 3 x 1/2 in. medium thin.

Butter.

Cream.

Tea.

DINNER.

Broth.	180 c.c.	1 glass.
Chicken.	100 grams	1 medium serving.
Baked potato.	100 grams	1 medium.
Tomato.	100 grams	2 h. tbsp.
Lettuce.	25 grams	3 leaves.
Olive oil.	13 grams	1 tbsp.
Butter.		
Cream.		
Tea.		

SUPPER.

Egg.	1	
Cabbage.	100 grams	2 h. tbsp.
Celery.	100 grams	6 stalks 4-1/2 in. long.
Onions.	100 grams	2 h. tbsp.
Butter.		
Tea.		
Cream.		

Allow during day:

Butter.	25 grams	2-1/2 squares.
Cream, 40%.	7 ounces	14 tbsp.

TABLE XXXVIII.

Protein, 71 grams

Carbohydrate, 60 grams

Fat, 184 grams

Calories, 2242

BREAKFAST.

Bacon.	100 grams	4 slices 6 in. long
Egg.	1	
Asparagus.	100 grams	2 h. tbsp.
Bread.	25 grams	1 slice, 3 x 2 x 1/2 in.
Butter.		
Cream.		
Coffee.		

DINNER.

Broth.	180 c.c.	1 glass or cup.
Steak.	100 grams	1 small serving.
Spinach.	100 grams	2 h. tbsp.
Carrots.	100 grams	2 h. tbsp.
Butter.		
Cream.		
Tea.		

SUPPER.

Egg.	1	
Lettuce.	100 grams	10 leaves.
Lima beans.	100 grams	2 h. tbsp.
Cauliflower.	120 grams	2 h. tbsp. +
Beef juice.	4 ounces	8 tbsp.
Bread.	25 grams	1 slice 3 x 3 x 1/2 in.
Butter.		
Cream.		
Tea.		

Allow during day:

| Butter. | 25 grams | 2-1/2 squares. |
| Cream, 40%. | 7 ounces | 14 tbsp. |

TABLE XXXIX.

Protein, 72 grams

Carbohydrate, 65 grams

Fat, 174 grams

Calories, 2170

BREAKFAST.

Bacon.	100 grams	4 slices 6 in. long.
Eggs.	2	
Bread.	25 grams	1 slice, 3 x 2 x 1/2 in.
Butter.		
Cream.		
Coffee.		

DINNER.

| Broth. | 180 c.c. | 1 glass or cup. |
| Squab. | 100 grams | 1 |

Lettuce.	25 grams	3 leaves.
Cucumbers.	100 grams	1 h. tbsp.
Turnips.	140 grams	2 h. tbsp.
Strawberries.	100 grams	2 h. tbsp. +
Bread.	25 grams	1 slice, 3 x 2 x 1/2 in.
Butter.		
Cream.		
Tea.		

SUPPER.

Fish (Haddock).	1 very small helping.	
String beans.	100 grams	2 h. tbsp.
Parsnips.	200 grams	4 h. tbsp.
Bread.	25 grams	1 slice, 3 x 2 x 1/2 in.
Butter.		
Cream.		
Tea.		

Allow during day:

| Butter. | 10 grams | 1 square. |

| Cream, 40%. | 7 ounces | 14 tbsp. |

TABLE XL.

Protein, 71 grams

Carbohydrate, 65 grams

Fat, 183 grams

Calories, 2257

BREAKFAST.

Bacon.	100 grams	4 slices 6 in. long.
Egg.	1	
Bread.	20 grams	1 very small slice.
Carrots.	100 grams	2 h. tbsp.
Butter.		
Cream.		
Coffee.		

DINNER.

| Broth. | 180 c.c. | 1 glass or cup. |
| Roast lamb. | 100 grams | 1 small serving. |

Baked potato.	100 grams	1 medium.
Lettuce.	10 leaves.	
Asparagus.	100 grams	2 h. tbsp.
Butter.		
Cream.		
Tea.		

Supper.

Eggs.	2	
Cauliflower.	120 grams	2 h. tbsp. +
Spinach.	100 grams	2 h. tbsp.
Bread.	20 grams	1 very small slice.
Butter.		
Cream.		
Tea.		

Allow during day:

| Butter. | 25 grams | 2-1/2 squares. |
| Cream, 40%. | 7 ounces | 14 tbsp. |

TABLE XLI.

Protein, 77 grams

Carbohydrate, 68 grams

Fat, 185 grams

Calories, 2315

BREAKFAST.

Bacon.	100 grams	4 slices 6 in. long.
Eggs.	2	
Tomatoes.	100 grams	1 med. tomato.
Butter.		
Cream.		
Tea.		

DINNER.

Broth.	6 ounces	1 glass.
Haddock.	100 grams	1 small helping.
Cabbage.	100 grams	2 h. tbsp.
Onions.	100 grams	2 h. tbsp.
Baked potato.	100 grams	1 medium.
Tea.		

Cream.

Butter.

Supper.

Cold boiled ham.	75 grams	1 slice, large.
Bread.	25 grams	1 slice, 3 x 2 x 1/2 in.
Peas.	100 grams	2 h. tbsp.
Lettuce.	25 grams	3 leaves.
Celery.	100 grams	6 stalks 4-1/2 in. long.
Butter.		
Tea.		

Allow during day:

Butter.	35 grams	3-1/2 squares.
Cream, 40%.	7 ounces	14 tbsp.

TABLE XLII.

Protein, 77 grams

Carbohydrate, 69 grams

Fat, 186 grams

Calories, 2328

BREAKFAST.

Bacon.	100 grams	4 slices 6 in. long.
Eggs.	2	
Bread.	50 grams	2 slices, 3 x 2 x 1/2 in.
Butter.		
Cream.		
Coffee.		

DINNER.

Broth.	6 ounces	1 glass or cup.
Steak.	100 grams	1 slice.
Turnips.	140 grams	2 h. tbsp. +
Lettuce.	25 grams	3 leaves.
Bread.	25 grams	1 slice, 3 x 2 x 1/2 in.
Cream.		
Tea.		

SUPPER.

Cold veal.	50 grams	1 small slice.

Parsnips.	200 grams	4 h. tbsp.
String beans.	100 grams	2 h. tbsp.
Cucumbers.	100 grams	2 h. tbsp.
Bread.	25 grams	1 slice, 3 x 2 x 1/2 in.
Cream.		
Tea.		

Allow during day:

| Butter. | 30 grams | 3 squares. |
| Cream, 40%. | 7 ounces | 14 tbsp. |

TABLE XLIII.

Protein, 74 grams

Carbohydrate, 71 grams

Fat, 176 grams

Calories, 2220

Breakfast.

| Egg. | 1 | |
| Bacon. | 100 grams | 4 slices 6 in. long. |

Parsnips.	100 grams	2 h. tbsp.
Butter.		
Cream.		
Coffee.		

DINNER.

Broth.	6 ounces	1 glass or cup.
Chicken.	100 grams	1 med. serving.
Squash.	50 grams	1 h. tbsp.
Turnips.	140 grams	2 h. tbsp. +
String beans.	100 grams	2 h. tbsp.
Baked potato.	100 grams	1 medium.
Butter.		
Cream.		
Tea.		

SUPPER.

Egg.	1	
Parsnips.	100 grams	2 h. tbsp.
Lettuce.	25 grams	3 leaves.
Cucumbers.	100 grams	2 h. tbsp.

Bread.	40 grams	1 slice, 3 x 2 x 1/2 in.
Olive oil.	13 grams	1 tbsp.
Butter.		
Cream.		
Tea.		

Allow during day:

Butter.	20 grams	2 squares.
Cream, 40%.	7 ounces	14 tbsp.

TABLE XLIV.

Protein, 75 grams

Carbohydrate, 71 grams

Fat, 180 grams

Calories, 2250

BREAKFAST.

Bacon.	100 grams	4 slices 6 in. long.
Egg.	1	
Asparagus.	100 grams	2 h. tbsp.

Potato (boiled).	50 grams	1 very small.
Butter.		
Cream.		
Tea.		

DINNER.

Steak.	100 grams	1 small serving.
Potato (boiled).	100 grams	1 medium.
Spinach.	100 grams	2 h. tbsp.
Cauliflower.	120 grams	2 h. tbsp. +
Butter.		
Cream.		
Tea.		

SUPPER.

Egg.	1	
Cottage cheese.	50 grams	1-1/2 x 1-1/2 x 1-1/2 in.
Lettuce.	100 grams	10 leaves.
Carrots.	100 grams	2 h. tbsp.
Bread.	35 grams	1 med. thin slice.

Butter.

Cream.

Tea.

Allow during day:

Butter.	20 grams	2 squares.
Cream, 40%.	7 ounces	14 tbsp.

TABLE XLV.

Protein, 99 grams

Carbohydrate, 101 grams

Fat, 225 grams

Calories, 2880

BREAKFAST.

Oranges.	200 grams	2 small.
Bacon.	75 grams	3 slices.
Eggs.	2	
Bread.	35 grams	1 med. slice.
Butter.		
Cream.		

Coffee.

DINNER.

Lamb chop.	100 grams	1 chop.
Peas.	100 grams	2 h. tbsp.
Olives.	50 grams	13 small olives.
Almonds.	50 grams	26 small almonds.
Bread.	25 grams	1 slice, 3 x 2 x 1/2 in.
Butter.		
Cream.		
Tea.		

SUPPER.

Salmon.	100 grams	1 average helping.
Salad:		
Lettuce.	25 grams	3 leaves.
Fresh tomato.	100 grams	1 medium.
Mayonnaise.	21 grams	1 tbsp.
American cheese.	25 grams	1-1/2 x 1 x 1 in.

| Bread. | 40 grams | 1 slice, 3 x 3-1/2 x 1/2 in. |

Allow during day:

| Butter. | 40 grams | 4 squares. |
| Cream, 40%. | 6 ounces | 12 tbsp. |

TABLE XLVI.

Protein, 101 grams

Carbohydrate, 101 grams

Fat, 235 grams

Calories, 3010

Breakfast.

Grape fruit.	100 grams	1/2 small.
Eggs.	2	
Bread.	50 grams	2 slices, 3 x 2 x 1/2 in.
Butter.		
Cream.		
Coffee.		

Dinner.

Chops.	200 grams	2 small.
Potato.	75 grams	1 medium or 1-1/2 tbsp. of mashed.
Lettuce.	50 grams	5 leaves.
Bread.	25 grams	1 slice, 3 x 2 x 1/2 in.
Walnuts.	25 grams	5 whole walnut meats.
French dressing:		
Oil.	26 grams	2 tbsp.
Vinegar.		

Supper.

Cold chicken.	50 grams	1 small slice.
Egg.	1	
Bread.	25 grams	1 slice, 3 x 2 x 1/2 in.
Celery.	50 grams	3 stalks 4-1/2 in. long.
Peach.	100 grams	1 peach.
Butter.		
Cream.		

Tea.

Allow during day:

Butter.	50 grams	5 squares.
Cream, 40%.	6 ounces	12 tbsp.

TABLE XLVII.

Protein, 99 grams

Carbohydrate, 126 grams

Fat, 228 grams

Calories, 3043

BREAKFAST.

Lamb chop.	100 grams	1 chop.
Eggs.	2	
Bread.	50 grams	2 slices, each 3 x 2 x 1/2 in.
Butter.		
Cream.		
Coffee.		

DINNER.

Steak.	100 grams	1 small serving.
Potato.	200 grams	2 small ones.
Cabbage.	100 grams	2 h. tbsp.
Bread.	25 grams	1 slice, 3 x 2 x 1/2 in.
Butter.		
Tea.		
Custard or ice cream, using part of cream, and one-half egg (extra).		

Supper.

Bacon.	100 grams	4 slices.
Egg.	1	
Peas.	100 grams	2 h. tbsp.
Beets.	100 grams	2 h. tbsp.
Peach (as purchased).	100 grams	1 peach.
Bread.	25 grams	1 slice, 3 x 2 x 1/2 in.
Butter.		
Cream.		

Tea.

Allow during day:

| Butter. | 50 grams | 5 squares. |
| Cream, 40%. | 6 ounces | 12 tbsp. |

TABLE XLVIII.

Protein, 101 grams

Carbohydrate, 150 grams

Fat, 292 grams

Calories, 3744

BREAKFAST.

Grape fruit.	300 grams	1 medium.
Bacon.	75 grams	3 slices.
Eggs.	2	
Bread.	35 grams	1 medium slice.
Butter.		
Cream.		
Tea.		
Sugar.		

Lamb chop.	100 grams	1 chop.
Peas.	100 grams	2 h. tbsp.
Lettuce.	25 grams	3 leaves.
Fresh tomato.	100 grams	1 medium.
Mayonnaise.	21 grams	1 tbsp.
Bread.	25 grams	1 slice, 3 x 2 x 1/2 in.
Butter.		
Tea.		

SUPPER.

Cold roast beef.	100 grams	1 slice (large).
Olives.	50 grams	13 small olives.
Almonds.	20 grams	
Cream cheese.	50 grams	1-1/2 x 1-1/2 x 1-1/2 in.
Bread.	40 grams	1 slice, 3 x 3-1/2 x 1/2 in.
Butter.		
Cream.		

Tea.

Allow during day:

Butter.	50 grams	5 squares.
Cream, 40%.	5 ounces	10 tbsp.
Sugar.	40 grams	4 h. tbsp.

Tea.

Butter.

Dr. Edwin A. Locke's book of food values has been of much value in making up these diets.

The following shows the successive steps in building up a diet for a patient who starved six days before becoming sugar-free:

	Grams Protein	Grams Fat	Grams Carbohydrate	Total Calories
Day 1	2	+	5	30

Day 2	15	12	4	189
Day 3	23	18	8	294
Day 4	36	30	11	471
Day 5	18	48	9	560
Day 6	51	44	17	688
Day 7	52	51	15	750
Day 8	46	51	19	740
Day 9	49	78	20	1008
Day 10	50	101	21	1230
Day 11	49	123	19	1422
Day 12	Starved because sugar came through			
Day 13	15	12	3	185
Day 14	34	32	10	478

Day 15   53   100   15   1208

Patient discharged with advice as to diet. The corresponding menus for the above are as follows:

FIRST DAY.

BREAKFAST.	DINNER.	SUPPER.
String beans 25 grams.	Lettuce 25 grams.	Lettuce 25 grams.
Lettuce 25 grams.	Cucumbers 25 grams.	Tomato 25 grams.
Coffee.	Tea.	Tea.

Protein 2 grams, Fat, trace, Carbohydrate 5 grams, Calories 30.

SECOND DAY.

BREAKFAST.	DINNER.	SUPPER.

Egg 1.	Egg 1.	Lettuce 25 grams.
Lettuce 25 grams.	Lettuce 25 grams.	String beans 25 grams.
Cucumbers 25 grams.	String beans 25 grams.	Tea.
Coffee.	Tea.	

Protein 15 grams, Fat 12 grams, Carbohydrate 4 grams, Calories 189.

THIRD DAY.

BREAKFAST.	DINNER.	SUPPER.
Egg 1.	Egg 1.	Egg 1.
Asparagus 50 grams.	Cauliflower 50 grams.	String beans 75 grams.
Lettuce 25 grams.	Lettuce 50 grams.	Celery 50 grams.

Protein 28 grams, Fat 18 grams, Carbohydrate 8 grams, Calories 294.

FOURTH DAY.

BREAKFAST.	DINNER.	SUPPER.
Egg 1.	Chicken broth 6 oz.	Egg 1.
String beans 100 grams.	Egg 1.	Egg whites 2.
Coffee.	Celery 100 grams.	Lettuce 75 grams.
Cream 1 oz.	Tea.	Cucumbers 50 grams.

Protein 36 grams, Fat 30 grams, Carbohydrate 11 grams, Calories 471.

FIFTH DAY.

BREAKFAST.	DINNER.	SUPPER.

Egg 1.	String beans 75 grams.	Egg 1.
Cauliflower 100 grams.	Lettuce 25 grams.	Asparagus.
Coffee.	Tomatoes 50 grams.	Tea.
Cream 2 tbsp.	Butter 1 square.	Cream 2 tbsp.
Butter 1/2 square.	Tea.	
	Cream 2 tbsp.	

Protein 18 grams, Fat 48 grams, Carbohydrate 10 grams, Calories 560.

SIXTH DAY.

BREAKFAST.	DINNER.	SUPPER.
Egg 1.	Broth 6 oz.	Egg 1.
Spinach 75 grams.	Chicken 50 grams.	Egg whites 2.

Butter 1/2 square.	Lettuce 50 grams.	String beans 75 grams.
Coffee.	Tomatoes 75 grams.	Cucumbers 75 grams.
Cream 1 tbsp.	Asparagus 75 grams.	Tea.
	Tea.	Cream 1 tbsp.
	Cream 1 tbsp.	Butter 1/2 square.

Protein 51 grams, Fat 44 grams, Carbohydrate 17 grams, Calories 688.

SEVENTH DAY.

BREAKFAST.	DINNER.	SUPPER.
Eggs 2.	Beef broth 6 oz.	Egg 1.
Asparagus 100 grams.	Scraped beef 50 grams.	Salmon 50 grams.

Coffee.	Cauliflower 100 grams.	Cabbage 100 grams.
Cream 1 tbsp.	Spinach 100 grams.	Tomatoes (raw) 75 grams.
Lettuce 25 grams.	String beans 100 grams.	Tea.
Tea.	Cream 1 tbsp.	Cream 1 tbsp.

Protein 52 grams, Fat 51 grams, Carbohydrate 15 grams, Calories 750.

EIGHTH DAY.

BREAKFAST.	DINNER.	SUPPER.
Egg 1.	Chicken 75 grams.	Egg 1.
String beans 100 grams.	Cauliflower 100 grams.	Spinach 100 grams.
Asparagus 100 grams.	Olives 25 grams.	Celery 50 grams.

Coffee.	Cucumbers 50 grams.	Lettuce 50 grams.
Cream 1 tbsp.	Tea.	Tea.
	Cream 1 tbsp.	Cream 1 tbsp.

Protein 46 grams, Fat 51 grams, Carbohydrate 19 grams, Calories 740.

NINTH DAY.

BREAKFAST.	DINNER.	SUPPER.
Egg 1.	Chicken 75 grams.	Egg 1.
Egg white 1.	String beans 100 grams.	Cauliflower 100 grams.
Spinach 100 grams.	Asparagus 100 grams.	Cucumbers 50 grams.
Celery 50 grams.	Olives 25 grams.	Lettuce 50 grams.
Coffee.	Tea.	Tea.

Cream 2 tbsp.   Cream 1 tbsp.   Cream 1 tbsp.

Butter   1 Butter 1-1/2 square.   Butter   1
square.   square.

Protein 49 grams, Fat 77 grams, Carbohydrate 19 grams, Calories 1008.

TENTH DAY.

BREAKFAST.	DINNER.	SUPPER.
Egg 1.	Lamb chop 75 grams.	Egg 1.
Lettuce 50 grams.	Spinach 100 grams.	Salmon 50 grams.
String beans 100 grams.	Celery 50 grams.	Asparagus 100 grams.
Cucumbers 100 grams.	Olives 25 grams.	Cabbage 100 grams.
Coffee.	Tea.	Tea.

Cream 2 tbsp.   Cream 2 tbsp.   Cream 2 tbsp.

Protein 50 grams, Fat 101 grams, Carbohydrate 21 grams, Calories 1230.

ELEVENTH DAY.

BREAKFAST.	DINNER.	SUPPER.
Bacon 50 grams.	Beef broth 8 oz.	Egg 1.
Asparagus 100 grams.	Chicken 75 grams.	Tomatoes 100 grams.
Spinach 100 grams.	Cabbage 100 grams.	Spinach 50 grams.
Butter 2 squares.	Cucumbers 50 grams.	Butter 2 squares.
Cream 3 tbsp.	Butter 3 squares.	Cream 1 tbsp.
	Cream (made into ice cream) 4 tbsp.	

Protein 49 grams, Fat 123 grams, Carbohydrate 19 grams, Calories 1422.

TWELFTH DAY.

BREAKFAST.	DINNER.	SUPPER.
Black coffee.	Chicken broth 8 oz.	Beef broth 8 oz.

Protein 12 grams, Calories 49.

THIRTEENTH DAY.

BREAKFAST.	DINNER.	SUPPER.
String beans 50 grams.	Egg 1.	Egg 1.
Black coffee.	Asparagus 50 grams.	Cabbage 50 grams.
	Tea.	Tea.

Protein 15 grams, Fat 12 grams, Carbohydrate 4 grams, Calories 185.

FOURTEENTH DAY.

BREAKFAST.	DINNER.	SUPPER.
Egg 1.	Roast chicken 50 grams.	Egg 1.
String beans 100 grams.	Asparagus 100 grams.	Cauliflower 100 grams.
Coffee.	Cabbage 100 grams.	Tea.
Cream 1 tbsp.	Tea.	Cream 1 tbsp.
	Cream 1 tbsp.	

Protein 34 grams, Fat 32 grams, Carbohydrate 10 grams, Calories 478.

FIFTEENTH DAY.

BREAKFAST.	DINNER.	SUPPER.

Egg 1.   Squab 100 grams.   Egg 1.

Tomatoes 50   String beans 100   Cold chicken
grams.   grams.   25 grams.

Coffee.   Cauliflower 150   Lettuce 50
               grams.   grams.

Cream 2 tbsp. Butter 1 square.   Spinach 50
                                   grams.

               Custard made with 1   Tea.
               egg, 4 tbsp.

               cream and 2 tbsp.
               water sweetened

               with saccharine.

                                   Cream 2 tbsp.

               Tea.

Protein 53 grams, Fat 100 grams, Carbohydrate 15
grams, Calories 1208.

Patient discharged with advice as to diet.

FOOD VALUES.

An estimate of the quantity or bulk of food may be of assistance or interest. There is so much variation in the size of tablespoons or what may be termed either rounding or heaping tablespoons that it must be remembered that we can only estimate. Patients who are instructed how to feed themselves on leaving the hospital are cautioned carefully to take about the quantity of an article of food they have been served while in the hospital when the diet is weighed. Any written advice is always given in quantities known to be *under* the carbohydrate or protein tolerance of the patient. However, if they will boil the vegetables and change the water at least twice, so much carbohydrate is removed that it is quite possible for them to obtain a comfortable bulk and still take in very small quantities of carbohydrate.

100-GRAM PORTIONS.

Asparagus—8 or 9 stalks 4 inches long.

Beans (string) (cut in small pieces) 3 heaping tablespoons.

Bacon—4 slices 6 inches long, 2 inches wide.

Cabbage (cooked)—3 heaping tablespoons.

Cauliflower—3 rounding tablespoons.

Celery—6 pieces 4-1/2 inches long, medium thickness.

Cheese—a piece 4 inches by 1-1/2 inch by 1 inch.

Cucumbers—12 slices 1/8 inch thick, 1/2 inch in diameter.

Greens (spinach, kale, etc.)—2 heaping tablespoons.

Lettuce—10 to 12 medium-sized leaves.

Onions—2 onions, size of an egg.

Olives—25 small olives.

Peas—3 rounding tablespoons.

Potatoes (baked)—1 small potato, size of egg.

Potatoes (mashed)—2 rounding tablespoons.

Sardines—28 sardines—1 small box.

Salmon—1/4 can (almost).

Tomatoes—2-1/2 heaping tablespoons.

Tomatoes—fresh, one medium sized tomato, 2 inches in diameter.

Bacon loses about half of its fat content when cooked.

Other Weights.

1 tablespoon olive oil	= 13 grams
1 tablespoon mayonnaise	= 21 grams
1 thin slice of bread (baker's loaf)	= 25 grams
1 medium sized orange	= 150 grams
1 peach	= 125 grams
1 medium sized apple	= 150 grams
1/2 small grape fruit	= 150 grams
1 medium sized lamb chop with bone	= 100 grams
1 medium sized slice cold tongue	= 25 grams
1 slice tenderloin steak 1 in. thick	= 100 grams
1 average helping of fish	= 100 grams

1 average helping of = 10 grams
butter

1 average sized egg = 50 grams

1 average helping of = 100 grams
cooked green vegetables
such as spinach, cabbage,
cauliflower, asparagus,
etc. (2 tablespoons)

1 average helping boiled = 100 grams
cereal

1 potato, size of large egg = 100 grams

> It is not true that all the vegetables weigh the same, but for the sake of simplicity in most of the diets it has been reckoned that two heaping tablespoons of any one of the "5%" vegetables weighs 100 gms.

The following food values are taken from Locke's Abstract of Atwater and Bryant's Bulletin No. 28, 1906, United States Department of Agriculture.

Fractions of per cents. have been left off in order to make the use of the table more simple, and the values given will be found quite accurate enough for clinical purposes.

Food Stuffs. Raw.	Quantity	Protein. Grams.	Fat. Grams	Carbohy drate. Grams.	Total Calories
Meat.					
ef	100 gms.	22	28		350
icken	100 gms.	32	4		168
con (raw)	100 gms.	10	64		636
Fish.					
h (average)	100 gms.	20	7		147
sters	100 gms.	6	1	3	46
Eggs.					
gs	100 gms.	13	12		165
gs	1 egg	7	6		84

ıtter	100 gms.	1	85		795
ıeese (merican)	100 gms.	28	35	2	448
ıeese (eufchâtel)	100 gms.	19	27	2	337
ilk (whole)	100 gms.	3	4	5	70
ilk (whole)	1 qt.	30	36	45	642
ilk (skim)	100 gms.	3	0.3	5	35
ilk (skim)	1 qt.	31	3	46	343
eam (gravity)	100 gms.	3	16	5	181
eam (gravity)	1 pt.	12	73	23	822

CEREAL
PRODUCTS.

tmeal ooked)	100 gms.	3	0.5	12	66
ce (cooked)	100 gms.	3	0.1	24	112
acaroni ooked)	100 gms.	3	0.1	24	112
ead	100 gms.	9	1	53	264
da crackers	100 gms.	10	9	73	424
ke (average)	100 gms.	6	9	63	367

VEGETABLES.

paragus nned)	100 gms.	2	1	3	30
ans (dried)	100 gms.	22	2	59	350
ans (string) sh cooked	100 gms.	1	1.0	2	22
ets (cooked)	100 gms.	2	0.1	7	37
bbage (raw)	100 gms.	2	0.3	6	35

rrots (raw)	100 gms.	1	0.4	9	45
uliflower w)	100 gms.	2	0.5	5	33
lery (raw)	100 gms.	1	0.1	3	17
rn (green)	100 gms.	3	1	20	103
cumbers w)	100 gms.	0.8	0.2	3	17
ttuce (raw)	100 gms.	1	0.3	3	19
ushrooms w)	100 gms.	3	0.4	7	45
ions (raw)	100 gms.	1	0.3	10	48
as (dried)	100 gms.	24	1	62	362
as (green, v)	100 gms.	7	0.5	16	99
tatoes (white)	100 gms.	2	0.1	18	83

tatoes veet)	100 gms.	2	0.7	27	125
inach	100 gms.	2	0.3	3	23
uash	100 gms.	1	0.5	9	46
matoes	100 gms.	0.9	0.4	4	24
rnips	100 gms.	1	0.2	8	39

The values for all the vegetables are calculated from the *raw* vegetables.

FRUITS.

Apples	(edible portion)	100 gms.	0.4	0.5	14	64
Bananas	(edible portion)	100 gms.	1	0.6	22	100
Blackberries		100 gms.	1	1	11	59
Cherries		100 gms.	0.1	1	15	71

Cranberries	100 gms.	0.4	0.6	10	48
Currants	100 gms.	1		13	57
Figs (dried)	100 gms.	4	0.3	74	323
Grapes	100 gms.	1	1	14	71
Huckleberries	100 gms.	0.6	0.6	16	74
Lemon juice	100 gms.			10	41
Muskmelons (edible portions)	100 gms.	0.6		9	39
Oranges (edible portion)	100 gms.	0.8	0.2	11	50
Peaches (edible portion)	100 gms.	0.7	0.1	9	41

Pears (edible portion)	100 gms.	0.6	0.5	14	65
Prunes (dried)	100 gms.	2		73	308
Raisins (dried)	100 gms.	2	3	76	348
Pineapples	100 gms.	0.4	0.3	10	45
Plums (edible portion)	100 gms.	1		20	86
Raspberries	100 gms.	1		12	53
Strawberries	100 gms.	1	0.6	7	38
Watermelons	100 gms.	0.4	0.2	7	32

NUTS.

Almonds.	100 gms.	21	54	17	658

Chestnuts	100 gms.	6	5	42	243
Peanuts (edible portion)	100 gms.	25	38	24	554
Walnuts	100 gms.	18	64	13	722

MISCELLANEOUS.

Chocolate	100 gms.	13	48	30	623
Whiskey	50 c.c.	43% alcohol			152
Lager beer	250 c.c.	4.5% alcohol			130

ADDITIONAL DATA.

	Protein.	Fat.	Carbohydrate	Calories
Bacon (raw) 4 slices, 6 in. long 2 in. wide	10	64		636
Bacon (cooked) 4 slices, 6 in. long, 2 in. wide	10	32		338
		to 46		to 468
Beef (roast), 1 slice, 4-1/2 x 1-1/2 x 1/8 in.	6	7		89
Egg, 1 medium size, 50 gms.	7	6		84
Oysters, 6 large	6	1	3	46
Butter, 1-1/4 in. cube (25 gms.)		21		195
Cheese (Neufchâtel) 1 cheese 2-1/4 x 1-1/2 x 1-1/4 in.	16	23	1	284

Cream gravity—"16%"), 1 glass, 7 oz.	5	32	10	359
Milk (whole), 1 glass, 7 oz.	6	8	9	136
Bread, 1 slice, 3 x 3-1/2 x 1/2 in. (30 gms.)	3	0.5	16	81
Uneeda Biscuit (1)	1	0.5	4	20
Rice (boiled), 1 tablespoon, (50 gms.)	1+		12	56
Oatmeal (boiled), 1 tablespoon, (50 gms.)	1+	6	33	$5
Potato (size of large egg), 100 gms.	2	18	83	$5
"5%" vegetables uncooked) 1 tablespoon			2.5	10

'5%" vegetables boiled once) 1 ablespoon			1.7	7
'5%" vegetables boiled thrice) 1 ablespoon			1	4
Grape fruit as purchased (1 small) 300 gms.	2		30	131
Orange as purchased 1 medium) 150 gms.	1		13	57
English walnuts (6 whole meats) 20 gms.	4	12	3	140
Almonds (10 small) 10 gms.	2	5	2	63
Peanuts (as purchased) 15 nuts	6	9	6	33

These are all approximations of the values. The vegetables lettuce, string beans, spinach, cabbage, Brussels sprouts, egg plant, cauliflower, tomatoes, asparagus, cucumbers, beet greens, chard, celery, Sauerkraut, ripe olives, kale, rhubarb, dandelions, endive, watercress, pumpkin, sorrel, and radishes can all be categorized as belonging to the "5%"

group. It will be evident that the value of 2-1/2 grams of carbohydrates for one tablespoonful of these veggies raw and 1 gram for the same amount three times boiling is not exact, but it is close enough for practical purposes given that these different vegetables contain between 3 and 7% of carbohydrates.